Stop Arguing with Your Kids

Stop Arguing with Your Kids

HOW TO WIN
THE BATTLE OF WILLS
BY MAKING YOUR
CHILDREN FEEL HEARD

Michael P. Nichols

THE GUILFORD PRESS
New York   London

Published by The Guilford Press
A Division of Guilford Publications, Inc.
72 Spring Street, New York, NY 10012
www.guilford.com

Printed in the United States of America

This book is printed on acid-free paper.

Last digit is print number: 9 8 7 6 5 4 3 2 1

Library of Congress Cataloging-in-Publication Data

Nichols, Michael P.
    Stop arguing with your kids : how to win the battle of wills by making
your children feel heard / Michael P. Nichols.
        p.   cm.
    Includes index.
    ISBN 1-59385-003-4 (hardcover) — ISBN 1-57230-284-4 (pbk.)
    1. Parent and child.   2. Child psychology.   3. Communication in the
family.   4. Listening.   I. Title.
    HQ755.85.N524 2004
    646.7′8—dc22

                                                            2003025018

Contents

PART III
Complications

Preface

Few things are more exasperating to parents than constant arguing from their children. The "Do I have to?"'s and "I don't wanna!"'s that turn family life into a battleground are familiar to every parent. Debates over everything from bedtime to chores to homework, TV, the computer, and curfews exhaust our patience and sympathy. In far too many households, ritual bickering uses up so much emotional energy that family life becomes something more to be endured than enjoyed.

While I don't need to tell you how aggravating arguing can be, I'm not sure we always appreciate how destructive this pattern is to children and their parents. Arguing undermines parental authority to the point where children who argue all the time come to see their parents as adversaries rather than figures of strength to guide and support them. All kids test their parents to see how far they can get, but, believe it or not, children need to feel that their parents are in charge. Constant bickering robs parents of their authority and their children's respect, and results in children feeling unappreciated and ashamed of their own initiative.

When your child looks into your eyes and sees a reflection of herself, does she see a reasonable person with legitimate feelings and opinions, or does she see a stubborn, argumentative brat? What's at stake with chronic arguing is nothing less than your child's discovering what part of her feelings are shareable and what falls outside the realm of the acceptable.

Kids who argue all the time come to feel like a burden. Why not? That's how their parents see them, isn't it?

Fortunately, there is a way to change course. It's called *responsive listening*. Responsive listening is a skill that enables parents to take charge of conversations with their children, not by laying down the law, but by shifting from the mindset of an opponent in a struggle for control to that of someone actively interested in the child's wishes and opinions. The point isn't for parents to give up their authority but to use it to hear their children out before making what is ultimately a parental decision.

If you picked up this book because you're tired of all the arguments around your house, I think you'll find that responsive listening can help. You'll probably be familiar with some of the concepts in this book, while others may be new to you. One thing I know is that responsive listening, when it's done sincerely, can make a big difference in all of your relationships, not just those with your children.

Responsive listening differs from familiar techniques like "active listening" in that the goal isn't merely to reflect feelings or paraphrase what your child says but rather to draw your child out, to listen, understand, and acknowledge the child's opinions and wishes. Responsive listening isn't a ploy to outwit children by pretending to understand how they feel. It's a way for parents to learn something new about what their children think and feel. When practiced regularly, responsive listening creates a shift in the parent–child relationship, resulting not only in fewer battles, but also in children beginning to open up more to their parents. After explaining the steps of responsive listening, I will show how to apply this skill in a variety of challenging situations.

You may find that it takes a little practice to make a habit of responsive listening, but you'll find it extremely useful when you do. Once it does become a habit, you'll discover that responsive listening does a lot more than cut down on arguments. By helping you tap into your child's inner experience, it will have a profound and positive effect on your relationship. Ask yourself, what percentage of the time do you feel that relating to your children is a struggle? How often would you say that your relationship is adversarial rather than cooperative? By making a conscientious effort to practice responsive listening, you can change that for the better. Surely that's worth a little effort, isn't it?

The five steps of responsive listening are straightforward and highly effective. The overwhelming response I've gotten from parents in workshops is gratitude for the remarkable changes they've been able to bring about with this approach.

Responsive listening means making an active effort to draw your children out, to invite and encourage them to talk at length about their feelings and point of view. When parents I've counseled don't get this, and settle instead for a perfunctory acknowledgment of what they think their children are feeling, I assume that I haven't explained it well enough. Fortunately, in workshops and therapy sessions, I have the opportunity to clarify this crucial step. As a result of these conversations, I hope I've been able to do a better job here as a writer in explaining exactly how to apply responsive listening.

Responsive listening will not, of course, put an end to all arguing from your children. You can't always prevent arguments. But you can cut down substantially on the number of arguments and the damage they do. As I explain later in the book, responsive listening can be a highly effective tool in undoing the hurt feelings from arguments even after they occur.

Among the topics covered in this book are:

- How to avoid getting caught up in arguments.
- A quiz to determine how argumentative your child is.
- How to short-circuit debates about chores, bedtime, siblings, who sits where, homework, TV, and the computer.
- Why children don't open up to their parents—and what to do about it.
- How to promote respect for parental authority.
- How to defuse arguments when you're out in public.
- How to resolve persistent arguments over the same issue.
- How to discipline without getting into an argument.
- Whining.
- Tantrums.
- How to tailor your response to your child's unique temperament.
- A quiz to determine how argumentative you are as a parent.
- Why teenagers find it easier to fight with their parents than to get on with their lives.
- Silent arguing.
- How to negotiate agreements that work.
- Why teenagers don't say what they mean—and how to translate.
- What to do when children play one parent against the other.
- How to predict and prevent toxic arguments with your children.

Many contemporary approaches to helping parents communicate with their children use one or more of the steps of responsive listening. I didn't invent the idea of listening to other people's points of view, nor was I the first to discover the value of separating feelings from actions. What I hope I have achieved is a simple yet powerful combination of these elements. The ideas presented in this book represent much of what I've learned over the course of many years practicing family therapy—and trying hard to improve my own ability to listen better to the people in my family. But if you try responsive listening and it doesn't seem to work for you, let me know. Write to me in care of the publisher. Maybe I can help.

Over the course of many years, I like to think I've become a better therapist. You learn, after a while, what works and what doesn't work. But if I've become a better therapist, I'm afraid I've also become a more impatient one. By the twenty-seventh time you see a family stuck in the same old rut, you tend to lose a little patience. Fortunately, in most families I find a cotherapist—one person willing to set aside blaming and complaining, and willing to take the first step by changing his or her own contribution to destructive family patterns. No matter what anyone else does, one person can always change the system. One person really can make a difference. Maybe you can be that person in your family.

MICHAEL P. NICHOLS
Williamsburg, Virginia

PART I

How Responsive Listening Works to Eliminate Arguments

CHAPTER I

Taking Charge of Your Children Without a Battle

Katie was an adorable seven-year-old with curly red hair. She and her mother had just returned from spending Sunday at the zoo and then going out to supper at Katie's favorite restaurant. Even though it was late when they got home, Glenda agreed to let Katie play one of her computer games for half an hour before going to bed. It had been an exciting day, and Glenda thought Katie might need time to unwind before falling asleep.

Half an hour later, Glenda bent over to give Katie a kiss and said, "Okay, sweetheart, it's bedtime."

"Mom, *please!* Can't I play Pokemon just a little longer? I'm not tired, and I don't want to go to bed."

"Honey, I'm sorry, but it's past your bedtime. We've had a long day and tomorrow is a school day," Glenda said patiently. "You know how tired you are in the morning, honey, and if I let you stay up past your bedtime you won't be able to get up and get ready for school." Glenda wasn't one of those parents who told their children to do things "because I said so." She wanted Katie to understand the reasons why things had to be done a certain way.

"I'll get up, I promise!" Katie pleaded.

"Now, Katie, didn't we have a nice time at the zoo today? And didn't you get to have a special Pu Pu Platter at the Chinese restaurant? Now I want you to be a good girl and get ready for bed."

"Oh, *please,* just a few more minutes. I'm almost done," Katie whined.

"Turn off that computer and get ready for bed!" Glenda snapped. Enough was enough.

"You never let me do anything!" Katie wailed. "It's not fair!"

Now Glenda was mad. "If you're not in bed in five minutes, young lady, you're going to be mighty sorry!"

At this unaccustomed harshness from her mother, Katie burst into tears and ran upstairs to her room.

Glenda resisted the urge to go up after her daughter. She was in no mood to try to smooth things over. Why, after all that she did for her, did Katie have to be so uncooperative? Why did she have to ruin what had been such a nice day?

As she sat there thinking, or rather brooding, Glenda was distracted by the faint sound of sobbing from Katie's bedroom. Guilt stabbed her. Maybe she could have found a better way to handle this. Wasn't there some way for a mother who loved her child as much as she loved Katie to avoid sending a seven-year-old to bed in tears?

Fifteen minutes later when Glenda went in to check on her, Katie lay still, pretending to be asleep. "Goodnight," whispered Glenda. No response. She bent down to give Katie a kiss on the forehead and felt her stiffen.

When she heard her mother's footsteps going back down the stairs, Katie fought the urge to call out "Mommy, come back." Her feelings were a jumble of anger and grief. Why couldn't her mother have let her have just five more minutes to finish playing Pokemon? On the other hand, she hated it when she did something that made her mother mad. Would your mother stop loving you if you were bad enough?

Martin, who was fifteen, had always been a responsible child, and so his parents had given him a great deal of freedom. He'd been allowed to take the bus downtown by himself from the time he was ten, and by thirteen he was earning money after school by baby-sitting and mowing lawns. So it came as a shock when he told his father that he and his friends were off to see a Pamela Anderson movie and his father said, "Isn't that an R-rated movie? I'm sorry, but you're going to have to find some other movie to go to."

Martin couldn't believe what he was hearing. It seemed absurd for his father to forbid him to see such a perfectly harmless movie. It wasn't as if he was planning to see a porno film.

"Oh, come on, Dad, all my friends are going."

"I don't care what your friends do," Martin's father said. "If their parents allow them to see R-rated movies without supervision, that's their business."

Martin doubted that his friends ever told their parents what movies they were actually going to see. But he didn't say that. Instead, he tried to convince his father. "What's the difference between seeing a movie with you and seeing it with my friends? It's still the same movie, isn't it?"

"That's not the point. I don't want you sneaking into movies and lying about your age."

"Who makes up those stupid ratings, anyway? Why should I be able to see movies full of violence but not ones with a little sex? There's worse stuff than that on TV all the time."

"I don't know, and I don't care." Martin's father was tired of his son's tendency to argue about everything. "You're not going, and that's final!"

"Oh, all right," Martin grumbled and went upstairs to his room.

As far as Martin's father was concerned that was the end of it. He never doubted that his son, who'd never given him any cause to worry, would respect his decision on this matter.

Up in his room, Martin couldn't believe that his father could be so unreasonable. Having been allowed so much latitude when he was younger, he wasn't about to let his father now, at his age, dictate how he spent his time with his friends.

What Katie and Martin demonstrate, each in their own way, is what happens when children argue with their parents. Sooner or later most parents are going to end up having the last word. But that doesn't mean that anybody ends up feeling very good about it afterwards.

According to her mother, Katie was "very strong-willed." That's one of the things parents say about argumentative children. Or at least that's what they say when they're in a good mood. When they're a little less guarded, parents say things like:

"She always wants everything her own way."

"He *always* thinks he's right."

"She knows everything!"

In fact, complaints about children's arguing rank right up there as one of the chief aggravations of parenthood. If only they'd do what we ask, at least once in a while, life would be a lot easier.

"Why do *I* always have to . . . ?"

"You never let me do *anything!*"

"Please, please, please!"

"It's not my turn!"

Do these protests sound familiar? If so, then you know how frustrating it can be to have to deal with a child's arguing.

How Bad Is Bad?

Do you ever wonder if your child is more argumentative than most? Maybe all children are argumentative. Maybe your child is more reasonable than most. Maybe not.

When I was doing research for this book, I advertised in the local newspaper for parents who were willing to be interviewed about problems with "highly argumentative children." You'd be surprised who showed up.

One father I spoke to considered his teenage son argumentative because the boy sometimes wanted to know why he wasn't allowed to do certain things. Several parents thought of their children as argumentative, not because the children argued with them, but because they didn't always do what they were told. On the other hand, I've spoken to several nice parents in my office over the years who seemed to take their children's lack of respect for granted, even though their children were outrageously rude and disrespectful.

To get some idea of how argumentative your child is, take the following highly unscientific quiz.

How Argumentative Is Your Child?

Do the following descriptions apply to your child:

    1—Rarely?   2—Sometimes?   3—Often?

_____ 1. When you have a disagreement, your child is willing to let you have the last word.

_____ 2. When your child challenges you, he or she may argue with your ideas but is usually careful to avoid attacking you personally.

_____ 3. When you're giving your side of an argument, you get the sense that your child is just waiting to respond rather than making an effort to understand what you are saying.

_____ 4. When your child realizes that you mean business, he or she will usually stop arguing.

_____ 5. When you make a point about someone or something, your child tends to make the opposite point.

_____ 6. When nothing else seems to work, your child gets very emotional to make an impact on you.

_____ 7. When there is an argument, your child has a tendency to go on and on, trying to prolong the argument until he or she gets his or her way.

_____ 8. If you give your child a choice of options, he or she will ask for something that wasn't one of the options.

_____ 9. When you tell your child to do something, he or she gets up and does it.

_____ 10. You find yourself battling with your child.

_____ 11. When you and your child argue, he or she actively considers the point you're trying to make.

_____ 12. Your child goes on and on if he or she wants something; won't give up; tries to wear you down.

_____ 13. Your child usually has to have his or her own way.

_____ 14. Your child won't take no for an answer.

_____ 15. Your child will bring up again arguments that you thought were settled and done with.

(cont.)

Scoring: Add the numbers you assigned to items 3, 5–8, 10, and 12–15. Then reverse the scores (change 1 to 3, 3 to 1, 2 stays the same) you assigned to items 1–2, 4, 9, and 11 and add this score to the first score.

What your answers mean:

- A score of 31 or over suggests that your child is very argumentative.
- A score between 21 and 30 suggests that your child argues about as much as the average child.
- A score of 20 or less suggests that your child is not very argumentative.

As I said, this quiz is not very scientific. It's really just a device to get you thinking about your child and your relationship. If your child scored low on this quiz, congratulations; it should be relatively easy to apply the suggestions I'll be making in the following pages. If your child scored higher in the argumentative range, you may have your work cut out for you. On the other hand, you may benefit all the more from the suggestions you'll read in the next two chapters.

"Do I *Have* To?"

Like a lot of familiar experiences, "arguing" turns out to be not so easy to define. Perhaps that's because the verb "to argue" has two very different connotations. There is one sense in which arguing isn't such a bad thing. "To present reasons for a point of view" and "to persuade by reason" are examples of the kind of exercise in logic that most parents would like to encourage in their children. There's nothing wrong with a six-year-old who presents reasons for wanting to do one thing as opposed to another or with a fourteen-year-old who tries to persuade her parents to allow her to do something with her friends. Such "arguing" can be part of a reasonable discussion in which parent and child learn to negotiate the gap between their two different perspectives.

But you didn't pick up this book to learn how to cut down on the number of reasonable discussions in your family. The second and more familiar sense of "arguing" refers to those annoying examples of children insisting on having things their way without respect for their parents' point of view. When children argue in this second way, it doesn't feel like a discussion. It feels like being attacked. It's unpleasant; it's frustrating. Arguing in this sense isn't an exercise in reasoning; it's emotional bullying.

The "Do I *have* to?"s and "I don't wanna!"s that turn everyday routines into a battleground are familiar to every parent. Sometimes it seems that children are happy only when they get their own way. When they don't, their protests trigger a barrage of arguments that never seem to get settled, just broken off to be resumed later.

The essential difference between arguing as part of a reasonable discussion and arguing as a child's insisting on getting his or her own way is that *argument-as-discussion* doesn't challenge the parent's decision-making authority, whereas *argument-as-resistance* does. Maybe we should call the reasoned give-and-take in which children express their opinions but don't challenge their parents' authority a "discussion" and reserve the term "argument" for children trying to get their own way without regard for their parents' point of view or for their right to have the final say. It's this second sense of arguing, when children defy their parents and insist on getting their own way, that creates so much friction in families.

Arguments, like the one Glenda had with Katie over bedtime, are upsetting to parents and children alike. By their very nature, arguments upset the bond of mutuality between parent and child, leaving them feeling like adversaries. Suddenly Us becomes You-against-me. *Why, Glenda wondered, couldn't Katie be a little more cooperative? Why, Katie wondered, did her mother have to be so mean?*

Although a certain amount of arguing between parents and children is inevitable, when arguing becomes a regular feature of parent–child interactions, animosity displaces harmony in the household. Recurrent arguments undermine a parent's appreciation of her child as well as the child's feeling of being taken seriously and respected by the parent. If seven-year-old Katie starts arguing whenever her mother tells her to do something, Glenda may find herself longing for the time when her daughter was little, when she looked up at her mother's face with wide eyes and nodded agreement with everything she said. It's a sad thing when parents start missing the children that were, instead of enjoying the children who are.

Fifteen-year-old Martin's argument with his father wasn't just about going to an R-rated movie. That was part of it, of course, but like all arguments with real feeling behind them there was more at stake than the subject at hand. Martin had a point about how the ratings system censors sex more than violence. But his father, not wanting to give in, refused to acknowledge this point—or the child making it. What also didn't get acknowledged, because it didn't get discussed, was the boy's feelings about being too old to be told what movies he could or couldn't see.

At what point does a fifteen-year-old decide that if he can't ever win an argument with his father, can't even get a fair hearing, he might as well start disobeying him on the sly?

No one needs to tell parents how frustrating arguing with their children can be. Nothing gets done without a battle. From getting up in the morning to getting ready for bed at night, everything gets bogged down in a litany of "Please, just a little bit longer"s, "Why can't I?"s, and "It's not fair!"s. Everything is subject to debate. Everything is a struggle. Some children, it seems, are never without an argument, even if rarely a good one. They resist and complain, they demand and protest—anything to get their own way—leaving their parents feeling alternately helpless and furious.

By being forced into arguments with their children, parents are brought down to the child's level. People in charge don't have to argue. They're the boss. Bosses don't argue; they command. If the arguing is chronic, the whole balance of parental authority is eroded. Parent and child become adversaries. It's not the way things are supposed to be.

The emotionality of arguments escalates through a series of actions and reactions. Here's eleven-year-old Lorelei's mother:

> "I try to be flexible, but if I remind her to do one of her chores, she'll say, 'But I'm doing *this* now. I don't want to do *that*.' So I give her time, but when I remind her later, she'll still not want to do what I ask. She objects to everything I tell her to do."

When her mother gives her choices—"You can work on your homework at the table or in your room"—Lorelei wants to do it some entirely different way. "But I want to do it on the couch!" Round and round they go. Lorelei's mother says, "I get sucked in. She gets very irritable, and I get caught up in that emotionality. Sometimes it turns into a shouting match. I lose control because she loses control." Sound familiar?

That's where arguments lead—emotionality, loss of control, shouting matches. By arguing, often at the most inconvenient times, children turn what otherwise should be good times into anything but. The whining, the protests, the complaining—from the very children you spend half your life doing things for—are as much fun to listen to as the blare of raucous music when you have a headache. But it isn't just the noise. It's the wheedling, the demandingness, the me, me, me mentality that triggers resentment in parents. Everything becomes a battle of wills. It's exhausting.

It can start with a simple request.

"Please turn off the TV."

"Time to get ready for bed."

"It's time to get dressed."

The child resists.

"Oh, please, can't I just finish this show?"

"I don't wanna go to bed. I'm not tired."

"What's wrong with what I'm wearing!"

It's this resistance that pits parent and child in opposition to each other. The child's persistence provokes a corresponding insistence on the part of the parent. The more recalcitrant the child, the more frustrated the parent. In the grip of escalating emotion, something unfortunate happens. Parents lose their cool.

Even the calmest parents become reactive in the face of too many arguments. Unfortunately, emotional reactivity leads to a battle of wills in which the only way for the parent to win is for the child to lose. There is another way, a way that allows both parents and children to emerge as winners—responsive listening.

Responsive Listening Lets the Air Out of Arguments

Responsive listening is a proactive technique that enables parents to respond to their children's arguments without getting caught up in a struggle. By listening, instead of reacting to their children's feelings, parents are able to remain in control of their own emotions—and of their interactions with argumentative children. Responsive listening isn't magic and, as we'll see, applying it sometimes takes patience and imagination, but it goes a long way toward putting parents in charge of arguments they once felt exasperated with.

It takes two to argue. The child's contribution is insisting on having things his way. The parent's contribution is countering this insistence. If one person insists and the other counters, the argument will continue until someone is willing to let go of trying to have the last word. During the time that a parent chooses to listen to what a pleading child has to say, there is no argument. Eventually the parent may have to respond to the child's plea with a yes, no, or maybe. But as long as that parental ruling can be deferred, there is no need for argument.

When a child says:	*An argumentative response might be:*
"Jesse came into my room and messed everything up!"	"Why can't you and your brother manage to get along for one day?"
"Somebody stole my hairbrush!"	"Nobody took your hairbrush. Maybe you just misplaced it."
"I hate you!"	"Well, that's too bad, honey, because you just can't. . . .
"I'm not going to wear braces!"	"I know how you feel, sweetheart, but the braces will help make your teeth nice and straight."

Here's how a responsive listener might respond:

"Jesse came into my room and messed everything up!"

"Boy, you sound angry!"

"Somebody stole my hairbrush!"

"Oh?"

"I hate you!"

"I really made you mad, didn't I?"

"I'm not going to wear braces!"

"Why not, sweetheart?"

When children argue with their parents, they are expressing their wishes—and asking for them to be granted. They aren't tired—and they want to stay up a little longer to play on the com-

Responsive listening works by separating the process of *expressing feelings* from a decision about *acting on those feelings*.

puter. They wish they could see a certain R-rated movie—and they want their parents to let them. Almost every argument has both of these components: an expression of feeling and a request. Unfortunately, parents get drawn into arguing with their children's feelings in order to justify not going along with their requests.

When seven-year-old Katie insisted that she wasn't tired and didn't want to go to bed, her mother responded the way most parents would: with an explanation of *why* Katie needed to go to bed (as though explanations were relevant to why children don't want to do what they're told). Here's how this argument might have gone differently if Glenda had used responsive listening.

"Okay, sweetheart, it's bedtime."

"Mom, *please!* Can't I play Pokemon just a little longer? I'm not tired, and I don't want to go to bed."

At this point, instead of explaining why Katie needed to go to bed, Glenda might have drawn her out about what she was feeling. "How's it going with your game, sweetheart?"

Probably Katie would have responded to that invitation by talking about what she was doing, and probably she'd still be anxious to convince her mother to let her stay up until she finished. If Glenda were to stick with responsive listening a little longer, she'd again resist the urge to explain and instead say something like, "You don't want to stop playing until you're finished, do you? Sometimes you wish you could stay up as long as you want, don't you?" The essential point would be to invite Katie to express her feelings and then to acknowledge those feelings.

In this case, assuming that Glenda didn't want to change her mind about bedtime, she couldn't really put off the decision very long. So, at some point, she'd pick up Katie or take her hand and walk her to her room, saying something like, "I'm sorry, honey, I know you wanted to finish, but it's bedtime."

Although Katie might feel a little better at this point for having her wish to stay up longer acknowledged, she'd probably still complain about having to go to bed. But instead of getting upset about this protest and arguing back, Glenda could see Katie's complaining as an expression of her feelings that again gives her mother the chance to listen and be sympathetic. "I know, honey, it's not fair."

In this example the argument is short-lived, but the child ends up feeling less bad. Yes, she has to go to bed, but at least her mother seems to understand how she feels about it.

When young children protest their parents' rules, their "reasons" aren't always relevant. Why does a child want to stay up late? Because she does.[1] Parents who insist on explaining why a child should clean up her room or go to bed when they say so create the impression that their decisions must be justified—and are therefore open to debate. The more their parents accept their feelings, the less children question the parents' decisions. When it comes to responding to their children's protests, parents should talk less and listen more.

> **How does a parent learn what to say in order to disarm a child's resistance to doing what he's told? The answer is that you don't disarm a child's resistance—you learn to accept it as a perfectly legitimate expression of the child's feelings and wishes.**

Things are a little different with teenagers. Fifteen-year-old Martin's argument with his father about going to an R-rated movie had ele-

---

[1] If this answer seems hard to accept, consider the following questions: What's your favorite flavor of ice cream? Why?

ments of three great themes of adolescence: the freedom to do what you want, the hypocrisy of authority figures, and the right to respect for your ideas. Martin's father could have used the principles of responsive listening by doing one or both of two things: acknowledging his son's points by saying something like "You may be right about that," or by finding a moment in the discussion to invite the boy to elaborate on his perspective, in this case perhaps about the double standard in movie ratings.

For example:

"Oh, come on, Dad, all my friends are going."

"Do you think our rules are too strict?"

Or:

"Why should I be able to see movies full of violence but not ones with a little sex? There's worse stuff than that all the time on TV."

"You may have a point there. Are you just trying to convince me to let you go to that movie, or do your really think there's hypocrisy in the rating system?"

As with Katie's bedtime, if Martin's father wants to forbid him to go to that movie, he's not going to be able to postpone this decision until later. Nevertheless, there's always time for a father to recognize his son's feelings about not being able to do something with his friends as well as his ideas about how movie censors are more intolerant of sex than violence.

In both of these examples, it's not hard to see how a child's feelings can go unacknowledged by a parent who is only trying to enforce a little discipline. It's also easy to see how the parents in both cases could have made their children feel better by listening to what they had to say.

Responsive listening won't make a seven-year-old want to go to bed on time or a teenager feel good about missing a movie with his friends. But having their feelings heard and acknowledged will make them feel a little less unfairly treated.

Sounds easy enough, doesn't it? If so, that because I've abstracted two examples in which it's easy to sympathize with the child's point of view—especially if you're sitting back reading about it, instead of being the parent-on-the-spot, backed into a corner by an insistent child.

Even nice children argue a lot. It's natural for them to push for what they want—and it's natural for parents to feel like pushing back. The idea behind responsive listening is that arguments won't escalate if parents don't argue back.

Some parents complain that their children argue constantly. These children don't just make an occasional appeal for understanding. Rather, they seem to resist everything their parents tell them to do. One reason resistance becomes a habit is that most children rarely feel listened to. Oh, they get to do what they want a certain amount of the time; but you'd be surprised how many children feel that their parents aren't very good listeners. The adversarial nature of interactions with "argumentative children" is fueled by the child's feeling that he or she has to fight to get a hearing.

Responsive listening cuts down on the chronic arguments that some children seem so adept at dragging their parents into, because it breaks the cycle of the parent saying one thing and the child saying another. As long as both sides keep trying to get their own point of view across—and neither is willing to listen to the other one—the cycle of arguing can only escalate until it ends in anger and resentment. When you practice responsive listening you avoid arguing about your decision by not discussing it. Instead you listen receptively to what your child wants, feels, thinks, and wishes. As long as you're listening, there is no argument.

CHAPTER 2

The Five Steps of Responsive Listening

Responsive listening is a skill that enables parents to take charge of conversations with their children, not by laying down the law, but by shifting from being an opponent in a struggle for control to an ally interested in the child's opinions and wishes. Listening responsively puts you in charge of the conversation.

The five steps of responsive listening are:

1. At the first sign of an argument, check the impulse to argue back with your child and concentrate instead on listening to the child's feelings.
2. Invite your child's thoughts, feelings, and wishes—without defending or disagreeing.
3. Repeat the child's position in your own words to show what you think he or she is thinking and feeling.
4. Ask the child to correct your impression or elaborate on his or her point of view.
5. Take time out to consider your decision—on minor matters by pausing before responding with your decision, or for more difficult situations by saying that you'll talk more about it later.

1. *At the first sign of an argument, check the impulse to argue back with your child and concentrate instead on listening to the child's feelings.* When

their children start to protest, most parents' first impulse is to explain or repeat their own position. To break that pattern before it escalates into an argument, take a moment of silence to remind yourself that you're going to respond to your child's feelings before deciding on the issue at hand. Don't even start to argue; take charge immediately by listening.

In order to really hear your child's concerns, it's necessary to suspend your own agenda, at least temporarily. It isn't possible to listen effectively when you're just waiting to respond. It may take a little extra time to hear your child out. But the active decision to postpone negotiation in order to explore your child's thinking is the first step in breaking the chain of argumentation.

"I don't want to go to Dad's house this weekend!"

"It sounds like you have strong feelings about that. . . ."

Because children expect arguments to focus on the outcome, it may take a little time for your child to learn that you really are interested in understanding his or her feelings. On the first few occasions you try responsive listening, your child may be impatient to get to a resolution. The ability to resist being drawn too quickly into making a decision begins with a conscious decision to focus first on your child's feelings.

"Do I have to go?"

"What's wrong, honey?"

The easiest way to avoid getting into debates is to anticipate arguments in advance. Before you tell your child to come inside for dinner or turn off the TV or get ready for bed, remind yourself that a protest is likely—and that it is an opportunity to practice listening to the child's feelings. By the same token, you can learn to develop a reflex to respond to requests first as expressions of feelings.

2. *Invite your child's thoughts, feelings, and wishes—without defending or disagreeing.* Let your child know that you're interested in what she has to say by inviting her to say what's on her what mind, what her opinion is, and how she feels about the issue under consideration. Then give her

your full attention. You might begin with a question that recognizes what your child seems to be feeling.

> "You hate to go to bed this early, don't you?"
>
> "You feel bad when you can't go somewhere your friends are going."
>
> "Sometimes you just don't feel like putting away your clothes, do you?"

But remember, you're not trying to guess what your child is feeling; you're trying to get her to talk about it. You're not trying to be seen as understanding; you're trying to understand. The overused expression "I understand how you feel" often shows less empathy than does saying "I'm not sure I completely understand how you feel. Can you tell me more about it?"

Even if you feel yourself getting impatient or defensive while your child is speaking, it's important to restrain the urge to respond until you've heard him out. Just keeping your mouth

Be sure that you hear what your child is saying, not what you expect to hear, and not what you want to hear.

shut and pretending to listen may be preferable to interrupting, but it isn't the same as listening. To really listen, try to appreciate what your child is feeling. Imagine how you'd feel if you were in his place.

3. *Repeat the child's position in your own words to show what you think he or she is thinking and feeling.* One reason children doubt that we understand how they feel is that we fail to let them know that we heard them. Silence is ambiguous. Repeating your child's position in your own words is the best way to let him know that you understand. Don't sum up what you've heard as though that should be the end of it, however, but rather let it be a means of inviting your child to elaborate so that you can *really* understand.

> "Let me see if I understand. Megan came into your room and started playing with your Legos. You asked her to leave but she wouldn't, and that's when you pushed her . . . ?"

Notice how this paraphrase is expressed with a question. The point isn't to convey that you already understand, but that you're trying to.

4. *Ask the child to correct your impression or elaborate on his or her point of view*. This step is directly tied to the previous one. I'm listing it separately to emphasize the importance of getting your child to elaborate on how she feels and what she wants. The point of responsive listening isn't to reach some conclusion—or to cut off the discussion—but to get your child to talk about her wishes and opinions. The longer your child talks the longer the cycle of arguing is avoided. The goal at this point is communication.

Don't be too literal. Children often exaggerate. Try to understand what your child is trying to communicate, even if he or she hasn't said it quite as well as you might wish.

"I think I understand what you're saying, but I want to be sure. Do you mean . . . ?"

"I'm not completely sure I understand what you mean. You're saying [paraphrase]—but I wish you'd say more about how you feel so I can get it straight."

5. *Take time out to consider your decision*. Sometimes, after showing that you understand your child's reasons for not wanting to do what you've asked, you may simply want to reaffirm your decision. The conversation now switches from understanding to making a ruling. At this point, any attempt to explain your position only invites further discussion. Just tell your child what you want him or her to do. "It's time for bed. Let's go." If possible, use body language to reinforce your decision. In the case of bedtime, for example, taking your child's hand and walking him to his room makes further arguing less likely.

Posture and eye contact are important indicators of whether you are open to debate. Looking away or even walking away can help make it clear that you aren't open to further discussion. If you want to see an expert demonstration of this, notice how good some waiters are at looking the other way when you're trying to get their attention.

"Sorry, I know you think it's not fair, but you'll have to be home by 10:30."

"I think I understand how much you'd like to have a puppy, and I agree that it would be a lot of fun to have one, but—I'm sorry—I'm not going to have a dog as long as we live in this apartment."

What I'm trying to illustrate in these examples is that after you've heard and acknowledged your child's feelings and it's necessary to state your decision, make it short and sweet. Don't justify. Your reasons may be debatable. What's not debatable is that this is what you have decided.

At times it may be a good idea to separate the conversation in which you try to be understanding from the one in which you announce your decision. Doing so makes your child feel that you are considering her position, and it gives you time to think over your decision with less pressure. After a child has, for example, explained her reasons for wanting a new bicycle or a raise in her allowance, you can say, "Okay, I'll think it over and let you know." Or, perhaps, "All right, honey, I'll discuss this with your mother, and we'll let you know what we decide." (Then be sure to follow up later, as promised, rather than letting it drop altogether.)

If at all possible, separate the listening with understanding part of the conversation from the part where you make your decision.

Questions Parents Ask about Responsive Listening

"Doesn't it make sense in some situations to state your decision first and then invite the child's thoughts and feelings?"

Sure, why not. The reason responsive listening cuts down on arguing is that it offers children a hearing for their feelings. They may have to end up doing something they don't want to do, but at least their parents have heard their side. Most of the time, the best way to do this is to listen to the feelings first, let your child know that you understand, and then say what you've decided. But if it feels right in some instances to say no first and then listen sympathetically to your child's protests, there's nothing wrong with that.

Suppose, for example, that Mom has to run back to the office to pick up an important file, and five-year-old Janine insists that she and her friend Daniel will be perfectly okay playing by themselves for an hour. Mom doesn't want to leave the children unsupervised for that long, and she doesn't have time to argue. So she simply says, "I'm sorry, honey, but Daniel has to go home and you have to come with me." Then in the car Mom can take the time to allow, even encourage, her daughter to complain about how unfair she is and so on.

It's not so hard to listen to your children's complaints if you accept that you have the right to make unpopular decisions. If you know that you are the grown-up, it shouldn't be necessary to have to convince your child of the logic of your decisions.

"How does responsive listening differ from other approaches that encourage parents to listen to their children's feelings?"

There are a variety of approaches that encourage parents to listen to their children's feelings, but most of them are designed to bring the conversation to a quick conclusion.

> "I understand how you feel, but now I want you to do what I tell you."

Responsive listening, on the other hand, is designed not to summarize conversations but to open them up. Even if your goal is to get your child to do what you want, getting him to talk at length about his point of view is the best way to put him in the frame of mind to cooperate. A perfunctory acknowledgment of a child's feelings usually doesn't work.

Thomas Gordon, who developed Parent Effectiveness Training (PET), suggests that parents can cut down on arguments with their children by expressing themselves in "I-statements."[1] Instead of saying, "*You* left your dirty dishes in the living room," a parent is advised to say, "*I* hate to see my living room all messed up as soon as you come

---

[1]Gordon, T. (1970). *Parent Effectiveness Training*. New York: Wyden.

home from school." Other "I-messages" might take the form of "I sure get discouraged when I see my clean kitchen so dirty"; "I'm angry that you've come home so long past your deadline"; or "I can't read when you keep crawling up on my lap." (PET works particularly well with small children and puppies. Husbands may need to be smacked with a rolled-up newspaper.)

According to Dr. Gordon, "I-statements" are hard to argue with. Instead of scolding a child—"You did this," "Why did you do that?"—parents are urged to say "I don't like it when you do that." The second message, Gordon contends, only tells the child how you feel, a fact with which he can hardly argue. Expressing yourself in "I-statements" may help cut down on preaching ("You should never . . .") and name calling ("You're acting like a selfish brat"). However, while using "I-statements" may be all to the good, as long as parents use this device to keep the emphasis on their position, rather than opening themselves up to their children's point of view, they still may end up perpetuating the cycle of arguments.

The technique of "active listening" involves paraphrasing what someone says before responding with your own point of view. Thus if a child says, "Guess what, Dad? I made the basketball team," the parent might respond by saying, "You're really feeling great about that!" Or if a child were to say, "For some reason boys don't seem to like me and I don't know why," her parent might respond with "You're puzzled why they don't seem to like you."[2]

The intention is to encourage parents to be more open to what their children have to say. The problem is that when "active listening" gets translated into simply summing up what you hear your child saying, the focus is on the parent's perceptiveness rather than on the child's expression. The emphasis in responsive listening is more on getting your child to open up and express herself than on your demonstrating that you understand what she is feeling.

The standard advice about accepting children's feelings usually boils down to saying things like the following:

"I understand, you don't feel like cleaning your room; but I want you to clean your room anyway."

[2]Both of these examples are taken from Gordon (1970, pp. 53 and 81).

"Okay, I understand; you wish you could play with your brother and his friend, but right now I want you to leave them alone and go play in your own room."

Such statements are an attempt to empathize with what children are feeling and as such they are an improvement on scolding and pleading. The problem with the usual formula—"I understand, but . . ."—is that it tends to close off the child's expression before the child has had a real opportunity to air his or her point of view. The problem is that "I understand."

When you're trying to empathize with someone's feelings, saying "I understand" is not very understanding. It implies that you already know what they're going to say. Since you already know what they're feeling, there's no further need for them to talk about it.

Imagine how you'd feel if you were worried about an upcoming presentation at work, and you said to your mate something like "Honey, you know I'm a little worried about how I'm going to handle that project I've been working," and he responded with a perfunctory expression of sympathy, "Yes, I know you've been struggling with that," and then turned back to what he was doing. How would you feel?

What PET and active listening have in common is that they help parents understand the important distinction between listening to children's feelings and letting them do what they want. My criticism—namely, that a perfunctory acknowledgment isn't the same thing as a sincere and sustained attempt to listen to what a child is feeling—probably applies more to the way some parents have applied these techniques than to any intention of the author of the techniques.

Actually, a more useful thing to say when trying to appreciate what someone is feeling is "I *don't* understand."

"I don't really understand how you feel; can you explain it to me?"

"I think I understand how you feel, but I'm not sure. Can you tell me?"

The difference between saying "I know how you feel" and "I'm not sure how you feel" is the difference between being willing and not being willing to listen.

I don't mean to split hairs. Trying to appreciate what your child is feeling is not a matter of saying this or that; it's a matter of listening.

When your child is upset, empathic statements like "Boy, you sound angry!" or "Gee, that must have hurt" should be an invitation for the child to say more, not a means of bringing the conversation to an end. Because listening to a child's upset doesn't come easily—especially when they're upset at you—there is a natu-

> **Responsive listening is more than a brief acknowledgment of your child's feelings.**

ral tendency to close off the conversation. Thus, even when parents try to be empathic, their tendency is to communicate "Okay, I understand how you feel; now let's move on." When a child is upset, that's not enough.

The point of responsive listening is *not* to get to the point where you can paraphrase what your child has said. The point is to get your child to talk. It's the talking—the communicative act of expressing feelings to someone who cares enough to listen—not the accuracy of your perception that makes a child feel understood and appreciated. Listening is, to a large extent, a strenuous but silent activity.

Why strenuous? Because to listen you have to give yourself over to the other person's need for your attention. If you've ever spent more time than you wanted to listening to someone's troubles, then you understand something about the pressure of being asked to serve another person's need for an audience. What makes it even harder to listen to a child who's arguing with you is that it's necessary to resist the emotional pressure to defend your position. The thing to remember is that giving in to your child's need to express feelings isn't the same thing as giving in to his wish to overrule your decisions. When it's genuine, responsive listening is a way around arguments, and a way inside your child's feelings.

> **Responsive listening isn't a gimmick to outwit children by pretending to understand how they feel. It's a way to learn something about your child's inner world of experience.**

If practiced regularly, responsive listening creates a shift in your relationship. Not only does it produce more cooperation, but the listened-to child also begins to open up more to his or her parents.

When talking with another adult, we may allow the other person to state their case, but then we make our own interpretation of what they have said. At worst, we are preparing our own response while they are speaking. This tendency to assume that we know what the other person is going to say is even more pronounced between parents and children. Therefore, it takes even more self-restraint for a parent to listen carefully to her child without assuming that she already knows what the child is going to say. Sometimes, of course, parents do know what their children are going to say. But it's important to remember that children need the experience of expressing their thoughts and feelings—and having them heard and understood.

The best way to counteract the tendency to assume that you know what your child is feeling is to summarize in your own words what you've heard, and invite your child to affirm, expand, or correct your understanding. Here are a few examples.

Most of us think we're better listeners than we really are.

> "Let me see if I understand what you're saying. You don't think it's fair that you have to go to bed before Ian. Is that right?" Here again, the idea isn't to close off the discussion but to invite your child to open up. For that reason, "Is that right?" can often better be expressed with just a question in your voice: "You don't think it's fair that you have to go to bed before Ian . . . ?"

> "You really don't want to have to finish your homework before you go outside. You know that I think doing it before you go out to play is the best way to make sure it gets done, but you don't agree with that do you? Tell me how you'd like to handle getting your homework done."

In both of these examples, the parent is making a sincere effort to invite the child to expand on her point of view. In the second example, the parent's invitation to hear what the child thinks goes beyond listening to the child's feelings, to being open to suggestions. As children get older it's often useful to encourage them to make suggestions, rather than telling them what to do and then fielding complaints. I'll discuss when and how to use this strategy in subsequent chapters. Here, I simply want to indicate that hearing a child's point of view shouldn't be confined to feelings alone.

The mistake some parents make is summarizing their child's opinions in a way that betrays impatience, lack of sympathy, or the assumption that they already know what the child is going to say.

"I know, you wish you could stay up and watch TV."

The tip-off to the inadequacy of this response is the punctuation. Punctuating your acknowledgment with a period suggests that you understand, and that's the end of it—"I already know what you think." A question mark, on the other hand, suggests that you're really interested in hearing more—"What do you think?" The same thing is accomplished with an invitation to "Tell me how you feel about it."

A child who argues is a child under pressure. Getting the child to express her feelings at length is the best way to release that pressure. The longer the child talks, the more she expresses herself, the more you listen, the more pent-up feelings are released. Following the release of her pent-up feelings, the child will calm down a little and become more open to hearing you.

The first few times you try to practice responsive listening, some children may presume that if you are willing to listen to their wishes, that means that you are willing to give in to them. That's why it's always a good idea to separate listening from decision making, if possible.

"I want my children to respect me. Doesn't encouraging them to say why they don't want to do what they're told foster disrespect?"

Some parents are reluctant to try responsive listening because they don't want to encourage the disrespect they feel that arguing represents. When children argue, these people believe, they are challenging their parents' authority. That's true. What's more, these people believe that the effort to be understanding of children's feelings, especially when they're arguing, is part of a permissive mentality that puts children's feelings above respect for their parents. That's not true.

The idea that listening to your child's reasons for not doing what you want encourages disrespect is understandable but misguided. Children learn very quickly the difference between being allowed to express their feelings and being allowed to do what they want.

A parent who is securely in charge

> **Responsive listening does not promote disrespect for parental authority.**

(or even decides to act that way) can afford to listen with understanding to her child's wishes, because she knows that the ultimate power to decide rests with her. It's insecure authority that insists on enforcing obedience by silencing complaint. We all act on this impulse once in a while. When we're tired, when we're upset, when we're in a hurry and one of our children starts protesting, we just don't want to hear it. But the parent who "just doesn't want to hear it" most of the time creates a reservoir of unspoken resentment. The silenced child may do what he's told, but his obedience comes at a price. He doesn't feel understood or respected and, consequently, he doesn't respect his parents, whom he sees as arbitrary and unfair. Children have great respect for fairness. The more you listen to them, the more they will listen to you.

> **The more you respect your children's feelings, the more they will respect your authority.**

"The idea of listening more to my children makes sense, but sometimes I'm too busy for arguments. Doesn't responsive listening take up a lot of time?"

Yes, listening takes time. But if you want to change your child's behavior, the effort required to do so must take priority. If you want to break the cycle of arguments with your children, listening responsively to their feelings is sometimes more important than cleaning the kitchen, going shopping, or even getting to a meeting on time.

> **Responsive listening takes time. But stick with it, because, by reducing the incidents of arguments, you will save time in the long run.**

The effort to take time to listen—even when you don't feel like it—pays off with an increased sense of understanding that sows the seeds of cooperation. If you really can't take the time to listen, say so, but talk to your child later.

> "Honey, I'm sorry, we really have to go right now. But I would like to talk to you later about how you feel about going to church with Nana and me."

Incidentally, it's not necessary to make a pretty speech. It doesn't exactly matter what you say when you're in a hurry. What matters is talking to your child later—not to explain your point of view, but to listen to hers.

"Should I try to use responsive listening all the time with my child?"

No. The point of responsive listening is to defuse arguments by hearing your child out rather than immediately countering his point of view. Thus responsive listening is most useful when your child feels pressured to say something, even if it's something you'd rather not agree to. Sometimes children make simple requests about which there isn't much to say, except yes or no. Inviting a child who asks for a candy bar before dinner to elaborate on his feelings isn't really necessary. You could, however, take a second to acknowledge the child's wish before saying no. "I guess you're hungry, aren't you? But we're going to eat supper in ten minutes."

One mother who was learning to use responsive listening wasn't sure how to respond when she saw her son doing a lousy job of washing the dishes. "What should I do, ask him how he feels about not getting all the gunk off the plates?" Well, no. And maybe yes.

If you need to scold (or "remind") your child about something, by all means do so. Responsive listening wouldn't necessarily be useful unless your child wanted to argue about what you were saying. On the other hand, if you have really good communication with your child, you might ask him—at some other time—how he feels about your wanting, say, the dishes to be washed so thoroughly. It may be hard to make such questions sound anything other than rhetorical, but if you can make it a real question, your child might admit that he thinks your standards are too fussy. What good will that do? By acknowledging such feelings, a parent is showing respect and giving the child a voice, which helps release the resentment that otherwise guarantees nothing more than grudging compliance.

Responsive listening is most useful when a child's feelings are stirred up. If your son or daughter were visibly upset and wanted to talk about something that happened at school, you'd listen, wouldn't you? It's just as important to listen when your child is upset about something between the two of you.

The most important time to use responsive listening is when your child is upset.

What happens if a parent doesn't listen to a child who thinks she's being unfair? Probably an argument, for one thing. If the conversation ends with the child feeling that the parent didn't listen, the child will be convinced that he was right: His parent isn't fair.

Now that you've been introduced to responsive listening, let's look a little closer at how it can empower parents by enabling them to avoid the emotionality that fuels arguments by bringing them down to the child's level.

CHAPTER 3

How to Head Off Arguments Before They Start

"It's time to get ready for bed, sweetheart," Ellen said.

Kirsty, age five, looked up at her. "Do I have to?" she demanded, pushing out her lower lip.

Ellen felt her stomach knotting. Lately Kirsty had been challenging her about everything. Ellen's solution was to try to stay calm and express herself as patiently as possible. "Yes, honey, you have to," she said, forcing a smile. "You know you have to get up and get ready for school tomorrow."

"But Paulie gets to stay up later, and he's younger than me!" Kirsty's voice was now close to a wail. "It's not fair!"

"Paulie gets to stay up later because he took a nap." Ellen's voice was firm. "You have more to do than Paulie because you're older." Why did she always feel compelled to explain herself to Kirsty?

"But I *always* have to go to bed first! Why do I always have to be the one to do *everything?*"

Ellen looked down at Kirsty, who was glaring at her angrily. Getting Kirsty ready for bed, which should have taken about ten minutes, had already consumed twice that. Ellen summoned a smile she didn't feel and took Kirsty's hand. "Bedtime," she said firmly. In Kirsty's bedroom, Ellen knelt on the rug to undress her. She undid the straps and slid off her overalls. Kirsty stepped out of the overalls and snatched them away from her mother. "I can do it myself!" she said, then flung the overalls into the corner.

"Those belong in the clothes hamper, young lady," Ellen said, getting angry herself now.

Kirsty stomped over to pick up her overalls and thrust them into the hamper. "Where's my pink PJ's?" she asked accusatorially.

"I don't know," Ellen said, "I think they're downstairs waiting to be washed." Why did everything have to be such a struggle?

"I want my pink PJ's," said Kirsty, her face tense.

"I'm sorry," Ellen said, "I didn't get a chance to wash them yet. You'll have to wear your Barney pajamas tonight."

"I hate those stupid pajamas! Why don't you ever wash anything around here?" Kirsty's voice was increasingly belligerent.

"Stop it," Ellen said warningly. "I've had enough of this. It's time for you to be in bed. Now put on those pajamas and get under the covers."

By the time Ellen finally got Kirsty into bed and the lights out, she was exhausted. Arguing with Kirsty made her feel shrill and helpless.

Kirsty argued about everything. Every night it was something different, as though a thin line of discussion was the only thing that stood between her and anything she wanted. Something about the relentlessness of Kirsty's arguing made Ellen feel increasingly depleted and unequal to the task at hand.

No one had told Ellen how it would feel to be a mother. She never imagined that children would be so fiercely needy, so demanding. Nothing had prepared her for these endless arguments. Before she had children, she had felt like her own person. Isn't that what growing up is all about? After living under your parents' roof for what seems like forever, you finally move out on your own. At work, people treated her with respect. She was someone to be reckoned with. How was it that at home she spent all her time arguing with a five-year-old?

Why Do Children Argue?

Why do children argue? Because they want something. (Sometimes it seems they want *everything*.) Children don't argue just to cause trouble. They always have an agenda—even if it's just to get some attention.

Kirsty wanted to stay up later. Her mother knew that if she didn't get her to bed on time she'd be too tired to get ready for school in the morning. But when you're five and you want to stay up and watch TV, the morning seems like a long way off.

Because children's agendas are often different from their parents', a certain amount of conflict is inevitable. In order to explore the world around them, children test whatever limits hold them back—including, guess whose? As much as possible, wise parents let their children learn from the natural consequences of their behavior. A parent doesn't really need to explain to a three-year-old that it isn't nice to pull the cat's tail. Fluffy is perfectly capable of explaining that herself, thank you very much.[1] The laws of nature are a good teacher.

Often, however, the limits imposed on children aren't a function of gravity or the *Feline Guide to Good Manners*. The consequences of a five-year-old's staying up too late are too far removed to have any immediate impact. Thus parents impose many of the limits children must endure because they understand consequences that their child doesn't, or sometimes because certain limits make things more convenient for the parents. Unlike the laws of physics, a parent's limits can be challenged.

The interesting question turns out to be not why children initiate arguments, but rather why their parents get drawn in and, second, how such arguments escalate.

Arguing with a parent's restrictions is one way a child has of experimenting with how the world works. Children don't argue to defy their parents; they argue to test the limits on getting their way. What could be more natural?

It Takes Two to Argue

Some parents resent the implication that arguing with their children is their responsibility. ("Why are the parents always to blame?") Other parents—perhaps more mothers than fathers—may be all too ready to believe that if their children argue all the time, it must be their fault.

---

[1]Parents who aren't willing to let children learn from the consequences of their own actions get entangled in their children's lives—like those parents who end up acting as alarm clocks for surly teenagers who never learn to take responsibility for waking themselves up.

One mother I spoke to wanted very much to know, "What did I do to make my child so argumentative?"

Of course, some children are more ready to argue than others. Argumentative children may be less flexible. They may be more stubborn. They may have trouble shifting gears. They may have low frustration tolerance. If you're a parent of such a child, it probably doesn't do a lot of good to worry about how your child got to be argumentative. In fact, such speculation may be part of the problem.

Thinking in Lines, Thinking in Circles

Questions about how problems get started are a product of what family therapists call "linear thinking." Linear explanations take the form of A causes B. This works fine in some situations. If your car suddenly sputters to a stop, go ahead and look for a simple explanation. Maybe you're out of gas. Maybe the frammutz has come unglued. If so, there's a simple solution. Human problems are usually a bit more complicated. That's why family systems theorists prefer "circular explanations."

Linear explanations are based on the Newtonian model, in which the universe is like a billiard table where the balls act unidirectionally on each other. While linear causality is useful for describing the world of forces and objects, it is a poor model for the world of living things, because it neglects to account for communication and relationships.

To illustrate this difference, Gregory Bateson, the progenitor of family therapy, used the example of a man kicking a stone.[2] The effect of kicking a stone can be calculated by measuring the force of the kick and the weight of the stone. If a man kicks a dog, on the other hand, the effect is less predictable. The dog might respond in any number of ways—cringing, running away, biting, or trying to play—depending on the temperament of the dog and how it interprets the kick. In response to the dog's reaction, the man might modify his behavior, and so on, so that the number of possible outcomes is unlimited.

The dog's actions (biting, for example) loop back and affect the man's next moves (taking the Lord's name in vain, for example), which in turn affects the dog, and so on. The original action prompts a circular

---

[2]Bateson, G. (1979). *Mind and nature.* New York: Dutton.

sequence in which each subsequent action recursively affects the other. Linear cause and effect is lost in a circle of mutual influence.

Circular thinking turned out to be enormously useful for family therapists because so many families come in looking to find "the cause" of their problems and to determine who is responsible. Instead of joining families in a logical but unproductive search for who started what, circular thinking suggests that problems are sustained by an ongoing series of actions and reactions. Who started it? It doesn't matter. You don't have to get back to first causes to alter a cycle of interaction.

When it comes to problems in our families, most of us aren't in the habit of thinking in terms of circular patterns.[3] It's only natural to blame others for our problems with them because we look at the world from inside our own skin. A teenager complains about his mother's nagging—but doesn't notice his own failure to respond to her requests. His mother complains that he doesn't listen to her—but isn't aware of her constant scolding. "Yes, but she wouldn't have to nag if he'd only start listening." "Yes, but he'd start listening if only she'd stop nagging."

He wishes she'd stop complaining. She wishes he'd stop ignoring her. Who started it? It doesn't matter.

There's a big difference between trying to figure out why your child argues and seeing the arguments as part of an interactive pattern. The first approach implies that your child is either willful ("bad") or impaired ("sick"). Either way, the implication is that you should try to change the child. But, as perhaps you've noticed, it isn't easy to change other people. The second approach—thinking of arguing as a problem to be solved, rather than worrying about how it got started—is far more practical. Once you start to think of family problems as part of a pattern of interaction, you can identify and change your part of the pattern.

To keep an argument going, children need help. Parents who argue back are their accomplices.

Not only does thinking in circles lead to a more problem-solving focus, it also helps you get past blaming and the resentment (or guilt) that goes with it. If you regard family arguments as the child's fault, then such labels as "stubborn," "bratty," "controlling," "defiant," and "resistant" will come to mind, and the idea of "teaching your child who's boss" will

---

[3]We may talk in circles, but we think in lines.

make perfect sense. But trying to
teach a child who's boss is likely
to fuel an adversarial pattern that
makes progress much more difficult to achieve.

> **Negative attention reinforces negative behavior—which in turn increases the negative attention.**

Difficult children tend to get locked in to certain behavioral patterns—but so do parents in response to that behavior. This kind of repeated negative interaction causes the difficult behavior to worsen.

"What's the Matter, Honey?"

As I said, kids argue because they want something. When they're little
and they ask for something their parents don't want them to have, their
protests usually take the form of whining, which may escalate into a
tantrum. Babies cry when they're hungry or wet or lonely. What else
can they do? (Children have few defenses, but they make excellent use
of those they do have.) The infant's cries of protest are the prototype of
all future arguing.

When hunger strikes, a baby hardly even knows what he's feeling.
Uneasiness grows. Then a painful feeling of emptiness intensifies as
hunger sweeps over him like a storm. The world gets dark, and he's
overwhelmed with a feeling of something going wrong.

The baby responds to growing waves of hunger with progressive
signs of distress. His lower lip protrudes. Then he starts to fret. Soon the
fretting gives way to fitful crying. If these cries aren't answered, they escalate into full-throated wailing.

The baby's cries are not some mindless reflex. Crying is not a passive experience. It is the baby's active and only means of coping with
distress. A child's crying, which can be so upsetting to hear, is a beauti-
fully designed signal to alert his parents to his distress and to compel a
response from them.[4]

It's easy to sympathize with a crying baby. (We were all babies
once.) Babies don't understand the concept of "not now" or "just a few
more minutes."

As infant researcher Daniel Stern explains in *Diary of a Baby*,[5] ba-

---

[4]Whoever came up with the first ambulance siren knew the power of a baby's wail.
[5]Stern, D. (1980). *Diary of a baby*. New York: Basic Books.

bies live almost entirely in the present tense. Thus their experience has a kind of all-or-none quality. Things are either lovely or lousy—in which case they urgently beseech their parents to make things better. A baby's cry doesn't feel like an argument, but that's only because we generally don't question the legitimacy of the need behind it.[6]

When a baby cries, her parents try to figure out what's wrong. Maybe she's wet. Maybe she's hungry. Why then do parents stop trying to figure out what's wrong, by listening responsively, when their children start putting their crying into words?

When children get a little older, their protests take on a more verbal form. Instead of just crying, a four-year-old might demand to know "*Why* can't I have a Happy Meal?" Now instead of just saying no, the parent's refusal is likely to include an explanation. "We don't have time to go to McDonald's. Besides, I thought you liked macaroni and cheese." The child disputes this, and the argument is off and running.

SIX-YEAR-OLD: I don't want to go to the doctor's. I hate Dr. Felch!

PARENT: That's not true. You used to like Dr. Felch.

SIX-YEAR-OLD: I *never* liked him. I *hate* him!

PARENT: What are you crying about? Don't be such a baby!

FIVE-YEAR-OLD: This oatmeal tastes awful! Why don't you ever buy anything I like?

PARENT: I buy lots of things you like. What about those nice apples we brought home from the country last week?

FIVE-YEAR-OLD: You never buy anything at the store that I like. All you get is stupid stuff!

PARENT: Apples aren't stupid. You used to love apples. What's the matter with you?

Somehow, once children get old enough to start putting their feelings into words, parents often take their complaints at face value. Instead of exploring their children's feelings—*Why* is a six-year-old afraid to go to the doctor's?—parents often remain sufficiently stuck in their

---

[6]Many parents, however, do struggle with the question of whether or not to pick up a baby who cries out of boredom or loneliness.

own perspective that they feel compelled to keep reiterating their own point of view rather than listening to what their children are feeling.

The spirit of responsive listening helps us relate to our children as children, not adversaries. Just imagine how different these two interchanges might have been if the parent's first response was to say, "What's the matter, honey?" and then to listen, rather than to argue.

Here's how this might look in practice.

SIX-YEAR-OLD: I don't want to go to the doctor's. I hate Dr. Felch!

PARENT: You *hate* Dr. Felch?

SIX-YEAR-OLD: Yes, I hate him!

PARENT: Why do you hate him?

SIX-YEAR-OLD: I just do, that's all.

Children don't always want to talk about their feelings. Some feelings are painful, and children—just like you and me—like to avoid painful feelings. On the other hand, there are times when children may not think their feelings are important enough to be taken seriously. There is no formula you can follow to get a child to open up. The thing to keep in mind is that you are trying to help your child release his or her feelings. Sometimes you have to probe a little.

PARENT: When was the last time we saw Dr. Felch?

SIX-YEAR-OLD: In the summer?

PARENT: That's right. Do you remember what happened the last time we went to see him?

SIX-YEAR-OLD: I had my allergy test.

PARENT: I remember. That wasn't much fun, was it?

SIX-YEAR-OLD: Dr. Felch said it would only take a few minutes, but it took almost an hour!

PARENT: Oh, gee, honey, I didn't know Dr. Felch said it wouldn't take long. That wasn't very fair, was it?

SIX-YEAR-OLD: No!

PARENT: Well, this time, we're just going for a checkup. There won't be any tests or any needles, and if you'd like I'll talk to Dr. Felch for you.

SIX-YEAR-OLD: No, that's all right. If there aren't going to be any more allergy tests, I guess it doesn't matter.

Jessica was clamoring to rent a video while Mom was trying to clean the house, mow the lawn, set the table, and make dinner for her friends, who were arriving in one hour. The more insistent Jessica became, the more irritated Mom's response. When Mom finally asked what's wrong and started listening to Jessica, it turned out that she was missing Mom's attention. After the guests left, Mom and Jessica sat down and played cards for twenty minutes, and both of them felt more connected.

What makes parents defensive in response to their children's demands is being pressured to do something they don't want to do, by someone they've already done plenty for, often someone who's being ungrateful, someone who's being selfish. At a certain point—say, after two or three no's—the child who keeps arguing is disrespecting the parent's authority.

Who's in Charge?

Arguments take place on two levels. At one level are the specifics. What time is bedtime? How clean is clean? How late is too late to be on the phone on a school night? Communications theorist call this level the *message,* to distinguish it from another, more subtle level, the *metamessage.*[7] The metamessage is an implied statement about the relationship between the speakers. If a wife scolds her husband for running the dishwasher when it's half full, and he says okay but turns around and does exactly the same thing two days later, she may be annoyed that he

---

[7]Bateson, G. (1951). Information and codification: A philosophical approach. In J. Ruesch & G. Bateson (Eds.), *Communication: The social matrix of psychiatry.* New York: Norton.

> The metaquestion in an argument is Who's in charge? When parents argue with their children they accept that question as legitimate. It takes two to argue.

doesn't listen to her. She means the message. But maybe he didn't like the metamessage. Maybe he doesn't like his wife telling him what to do as though she were his mother.

Arguing implies a relationship of equals. If you are firmly in charge, you can listen to complaints or demands without feeling the need to argue. You feel free to listen because you know you have the final say.

Parents who end up arguing with their children may not start out with any lack of confidence in their authority. They know they're in charge; they choose to explain their position because they're trying to be fair and respectful. Unfortunately, the process of explaining can convey to a child that the final decision depends on whether he accepts the explanation. If he can successfully challenge his parents' explanation, the child thinks, then he won't have to do what they say.

Explanations are complicated and, as we'll see later, the need for parents to explain their decisions depends on how old their children are. But regardless of a child's age, explanations in response to rhetorical questions—"*Why* do I have to go to bed?"—only invite further debate.

It's important to keep in mind that the message we intend to convey has to pass through two filters: our ability to express ourselves and the listener's ability to grasp what we're trying to communicate. The mother who responds to her son's protests by explaining the reasons for her decision may intend to convey: "You have to do what I say, and this is why I made this decision." But the boy who is arguing not to do what he is told isn't really interested in explanations; he just doesn't want to do what he's told. In this atmosphere, he will respond to his mother's explanations as an invitation to debate. The only time a child is likely to really hear an explanation is when the question of what has to be done has already been settled—stated *and* accepted.

When I was a newly minted assistant professor I dreaded meeting with students who came to my office to question their exam grades. Because I felt the need to justify my grading, these discussions often turned into arguments. The student would say something accusatory like "I don't think it's fair to take off five points just because I left out one little thing." I'd get defensive and say something snippy like "If you came to class more often you'd know that I emphasized that point." Then the student would get angry and maybe try one more challenge, until eventually I'd say something peremptory like "I'm sorry you don't like your grade, but that's the way it is." Eventually, I decided that if I'd done my grading carefully, I didn't have to change it, and therefore I could listen—with genuine sympathy—to the students' complaints, knowing that I had already decided the grade fairly. I stopped dreading these meetings and, in fact, came to look on them as an opportunity to find out what the students were feeling. I still rarely change a grade on an exam, but most of my disgruntled students now leave these meetings feeling better that at least I listened seriously to the feelings behind their complaints.

There were two things I had to learn in order to stop being defensive and start listening. The first was to develop a reflex to respond to complaints with an invitation for protesting students to explain their thinking—"Tell me more about what you think." Everyone gets defensive when provoked. The trick is to avoid getting caught off guard. If a therapist can learn to make a habit of saying "Why do you ask?" in response to personal questions, a teacher can learn to make a habit of saying "You don't think it's fair?" in response to a student's complaints.

The second thing I had to learn was, frankly, much harder. I had to learn to really take an interest in the students' point of view. I started out as the kind of teacher who was more interested in the subject matter than the students. When I was young, I related to students primarily as an audience. That's not easy to admit, but that's the way it was. Only gradually, and especially now that my own children are out of the house, did I start to think of teaching more as interacting with the students than as standing in front of them giving brilliant lectures. It should be a lot easier for parents, who don't have to learn to love their children, to be interested in their feelings. Don't lecture; listen.

When children argue, they're expressing their feelings and asking for something. They don't want to go to bed (they might miss something). They don't feel like cleaning their rooms (they'd rather be outside playing). It's natural for parents to resist these protests and demands. They're concerned with the outcome of these discussions—what eventually gets done. Unfortunately, that often means neglecting the process—whether or not a disappointed child at least feels that her parents respect her feelings.

We really do want them to go to bed and clean their rooms (not necessarily in that order). But giving in to the impulse to argue back brings the parent down to the child's level and leads to more arguing.

Here is a list of things children say that trigger a parent's impulse to argue back:

Child's protest	Parent's argumentative response
"It's not fair!"	"Yes, it is fair."
"Why can't I watch this program?"	"Because it's too violent."
"But all my friends are going to this party!"	"I don't care what your friends' parents let them do. You're not going, and that's final."

What do these parental responses have in common? In terms of their impact on the child, each one of these replies could be replaced with one phrase: "You're wrong." When someone argues back, the metamessage is always the same: I'm right, and you're wrong.

Here's how a parent who practices responsive listening might respond to these same protests.

Child's protest	Parent's receptive response
"It's not fair!"	"Why do you think it's unfair?"
"Why can't I watch this program?"	"You really want to watch this program, don't you?"
"But all my friends are going to this party!"	"Do you feel shut out when you're not allowed to do something your friends are doing?"

You can probably improve on some of those responses. The point is to avoid arguing back, and, instead, to open the door for your child to express his point of view. Children are never wrong about what they're feeling. But parents don't really hear what their children are feeling when they get defensive and start arguing back.

Some of what children say when they're invited to explain their wishes is fairly obvious. "Yes, I really, really want to watch this show!" But children sometimes have reasons for what they're feeling that aren't obvious. Maybe your child wants to watch a particular TV show because when all of his friends talk about the show he feels left out.

Maybe his teacher mentioned the show in class. Maybe your child feels that some restriction is unfair because he sees you doing the thing he wants to do yourself, or maybe his father or stepmother lets him do it.

Here's how one of the previous examples might play out.

CHILD: Why can't I watch this program?

PARENT: You really want to watch this program, don't you?

CHILD: Yes.

Just because a parent may be willing to explore a child's wishes doesn't mean that the child is eager to discuss them. In a case like this one most children just want to watch their programs; they're not interested in justifying their reasons. They're focused on the outcome. A parent who's interested in opening up the child's feelings may have to use some ingenuity.

PARENT: Isn't it mostly just a lot of killings?

CHILD: No. It's a whole story about a modern-day Mafia family. There are some killings, but most of it isn't about that.

PARENT: I thought the Mafia went out of business after John Gotti went to prison.

CHILD: Uh-uh. They're still in business, especially in New Jersey. They run the garbage business.

PARENT: I didn't know that.

At this point, even though the parent has demonstrated openness to learning about the child's interests, a decision still has to be made. One possibility would be for the parent simply to say no.

PARENT: I can see that there's more to this program than I thought, but I'm sorry, I just won't allow you to watch anything that violent.

Another possibility would be for the parent to watch the program with the child.

PARENT: I'll tell you what. I'll
record tonight's episode,
and tomorrow I'll watch it
with you. If there are violent scenes that I don't
think you should watch, I
will fast-forward past them.

Reacting defensively to the instrumental part of a child's message without acknowledging the feelings behind it is what turns discussions into arguments.

CHILD: Oh, all right.

When Is an Argument Not an Argument?

We used to have a little gray-and-white cat named Tina, who meowed
all the time. I like cats, but the constant meowing was annoying. One
day when she heard me fussing at Tina for
meowing, my wife said, "She's talking."
What a revelation! Of course she was talking. (Well, you know what I mean.) My
problem was that I saw Tina's meowing
only as an annoyance. I saw her as complaining, and I wanted her to
stop. Have you ever tried to make a cat stop meowing? It's about as
easy as trying to make a child stop arguing.

When is an argument not an argument? When you don't argue back.

How did I get Tina to stop "arguing"? First by seeing if she wanted
something that I didn't mind doing for her. If she meowed at the door,
I'd let her out. If she meowed by the foot of my chair, I'd pick her up
and pet her. If she didn't seem to want anything, or, more likely, I
couldn't figure out what it was, I just let her "talk."

If Tina were a child, I could have done more than just let her talk.
I could have let her know that I was interested in what she had to say. I
could have invited her to say more. I could have been more tolerant. I
could have let her know that her feelings were legitimate (except those
about her designs on my dinner). We could have communicated.

My problem with Tina was that my impulse was to control her—
not just her behavior, like sharpening her claws on the couch, but her
meowing, her only means of expression. Parents who make the mistake
of trying to control their children's protests end up making arguments
worse.

When it comes to the relationship between parents and children, there is a fundamental paradox between authority and control: The best way to maintain your authority is not to squander it, not to try to control too much of your children's behavior. Trying to control your child's right to express herself is trying to control too much. Take it from me, the big-shot psychologist who used to lose arguments with a small cat.

The act of listening requires letting go. That isn't always easy. A parent may have trouble letting go of the conversation with an argumentative child for fear that doing so will mean losing control of the outcome. Nothing could be further from the truth. Suspending control does not mean losing control—though that seems to be precisely what many parents are afraid of. Otherwise, why do they insist on countering every one of their child's arguments, when a simple acknowledgment of what the child is saying would be the first step toward mutual understanding? It's as though saying "I understand" meant "I surrender." When a parent's fear of not being respected is so strong that he or she doesn't respect the child's right to disagree, it becomes a self-fulfilling prophecy.

One reason children keep arguing is that their parents don't acknowledge their feelings. Parents whose first impulse is to insist often end up trying to make the child wrong in order for them to be right.

> "Why do *I* always have to take the garbage out? How come Ryan never has to do anything around here? It's not fair!"
>
> "That's not true! Stop complaining all the time!"

Sometimes parents don't acknowledge their children's feelings because they don't want them to feel bad. So instead of listening, they offer "reassurance"—a much overrated commodity.

What do children feel when their parents insist by making them wrong? That their feelings don't count. That trying to express themselves is a waste of time, because their parents don't listen.

> "What's wrong with me? Terri used to like me, but

now she doesn't any more. She never comes over here any more, and if I go over to her house, she's always playing with Carin. I hate both of them!"

"There's nothing wrong with you, and I'm sure Terri still likes you. Don't worry, things will work out."

When we tell our kids not to worry, the metamessage is that we don't want to hear it. Their worry upsets us, and so we try to be helpful by telling them that things will work out. Maybe they will, but reassuring someone by telling them not to feel what they're feeling isn't very reassuring.

Hard as it is for parents to listen to their children's fears and worries about other people, it's much harder to listen to their complaints about them. But it isn't just that their children's arguments challenge their authority that makes parents defensive, it's the *way* that challenge is expressed.

Don't Lose Your Cool

If conflicting agendas are what motivate arguments, what fuels them is emotionality. When your children don't want to do what they're told, they don't usually say so calmly.

"I say, Mater, I know it's bedtime and all that, but how about another spot of cocoa before I toddle off?" Yeah, right.

Children are fierce little engines of desire. Their entreaties are packed with emotional urgency. They spell out their wishes with capital letters and exclamation points. When they want something, they REALLY, REALLY want it!!

"*Please, please,* can't I stay up to watch *Buffy?*"

"I hate that stupid Mrs. Rogers! I'm never going back to that class!"

"Why can't I go to the concert? Everybody else is going. I'll be home by midnight, I promise!"

According to argumentative children, their parents are ALWAYS making them do stuff they don't want to do. Their parents NEVER let them have any fun.

"You *never* let me go anywhere. *It's not fair!*"

"Why do I have to take out the garbage right now? You *always* make me do things when I'm busy doing something else!"

Some combination of the child's demandingness and the parent's frustration triggers an emotional counterresponse of anger and resentment. The more reactive parents become, the less constructive their response to their children tends to be.

It's hard to listen to a crying baby. The crying radiates distress, making parents want to do something to make it stop, making strangers in a restaurant want parents to do something to make it stop. When older children start putting their upset into words, some of that same emotional contagion occurs. The child's arguing upsets the parents, makes them want to do something to make it stop. The "it" they want to make stop is as much their own distress as the child's.

Even the most self-possessed parents are prone to overreact when their children push the right buttons.

The emotional reactivity triggered in parents by their children's arguing takes a variety of forms: anger, guilt, defensiveness, frustration, resentment, exasperation. The common denominator is a tendency to react without thinking. According to family therapist Murray Bowen, this tendency to react without thinking when members of our families do what they do to provoke us is what makes us get into shouting matches or avoid personal conversations, or even contact, with certain family members.[8] Emotional reactivity has the same effect on most of us that kryptonite has on Superman.

What Bowen advises as the antidote to emotional reactivity, in case anyone should hazard a visit to their home planet, is planning in advance to make a calm response to whatever predictably upsets you. Your relatives don't have any tricks up their sleeve; they do what they always do. So, instead of waiting to be thrown off guard by your fa-

---

[8]Kerr, M. E., & Bowen, M. (1988). *Family evaluation.* New York: Norton.

ther's criticism or your mother's evasiveness, prepare yourself to respond without getting emotional. A joking comment may enable you to remain calm better than trying to set the other person straight.

> "Thanks, Dad, I can always count on you for some words of wisdom."

> "Gee, that was close, Mom, you almost committed yourself."

The same solution—planning a calm response—enables parents to avoid becoming emotionally reactive when their children argue. The bad news is that it's hard not to get thrown off guard when children argue at inopportune times. The good news is that you can arm yourself against reacting emotionally by developing the habit of responsive listening.

Here's an example from a friend.

> "On the first day of summer camp Zoe seemed excited. As we got closer to the school, she began to say over and over, 'I'm not going, I'm not going.' I wasn't expecting this. The night before she had been so excited that she had trouble falling asleep, and that morning she chose to have her hair in pigtails, because that's her choice for 'first days' of everything.
>
> "Zoe is slow to warm up and cautious, and she always seems to know her own mind. So we as parents are always on our toes. But somehow her last-minute resistance caught me off guard. I started to respond to her with an explanation. 'Well, honey, you know this is your first day and you have to go, and I'll walk you to the class.' All the while I was thinking, *She has to start camp today, otherwise how will I finish this project that's due tomorrow?*
>
> "The more I explained, the more tightly Zoe clung to the seatbelt so that I couldn't unbuckle her.
>
> "Then I remembered: 'Stop explaining and listen for the feeling.' So I said, 'I know sometimes you can have mixed up feelings like you don't want to go but you do want to go at the same time. Is that how you feel now?'
>
> "There was a pause. Zoe didn't say anything. Then she un-

buckled herself, got out of the car, and walked up the ramp to the school. I got out and followed her inside. Less than ten minutes later, Zoe kissed me and said, 'Goodbye, Mommy, I'll see you later.'

"There was little or no follow-up discussion, once I'd taken the time to talk to Zoe about what she was feeling. Maybe, in the process, I was dealing with my own separation anxiety as well!

"I don't see responsive listening as a magical cure for arguments. It takes a lot of effort, and I'm already pretty stressed out most of the time. But when I do make the effort it usually seems to pay off."

When children argue, it isn't just their requests that you have to deal with, it's the emotional pressure with which they come at you. The emotionality of their children's demands makes parents feel backed into a corner. When you're pushed hard enough, the natural impulse is to push back. But arguments aren't just a matter of pressure and counterpressure. When children pressure their parents, they go at it in an urgent, insistent manner. Argumentative children don't just push their parents' buttons; they hammer them. That emotionality is infectious.

Laura's fourteen-year-old son, Vernon, argues every time she reminds him to do something.

"Why do I have to wash the dishes *now*?" he says.

"I'm busy now," he says. "I'll do my homework later," he says.

"I don't want to go to soccer practice tonight," he says.

With Vernon, everything is a struggle. But what really drives Laura crazy is his whining.

"The constant arguing is bad enough, but when he starts whining in that high-pitched voice of his, I can't stand it. That's when I start yelling back at him."

Overreacting to a stubborn child isn't a sign of some flaw in a parent's character. Today's accelerated family lives impose a hectic, pressured quality on our daily activities and undermine our tolerance for interruptions and delays. It's one thing for a child to argue about what she's going to wear to school tomorrow. It's far more aggravating when the same argument erupts when you're late for work and the school bus is due in ten minutes. Anxiety feeds on pressure.

When you're in a hurry, an argumentative child ties your shoelaces together.

Reacting emotionally to a child's protests is what turns discussions into arguments. It's hard enough to reason with a demanding child. It's almost impossible when you lose your cool.

A parent's ability to stay in charge rests on how successfully he or she resists the pressure to react emotionally to the child's pressure. The simple but sometimes herculean act of not becoming reactive empowers parents to remain in control during arguments with their children, no matter what the pressure. It's simple, right? Just don't get upset.

The usual advice to people who lose control of their feelings is to learn to practice self-restraint. The trouble with trying not to react is that it's hard to concentrate on the negative. Instead of *not* getting defensive, concentrate on listening. If you want to react less impulsively, listen more deliberately.

Are there any tricks to help parents learn to substitute listening rather than reacting to their children's provocation? I don't think so. It just takes practice. It might help to remember that at least some part of that angry toddler or sulking adolescent will always be that sweet little baby you once held in your arms.

To avoid reacting emotionally when your child starts arguing, make responsive listening a reflex. As long as you're making a deliberate effort to listen, you're in charge—of the situation, and of your own emotions.

Break the discussion into two parts: First help your child express his or her feelings, as fully as possible. Second, and later if possible, make your decision about the issue at hand. If postponing your decision isn't practical, practice the Ten Second Pause. If you have to say yes, no, or maybe immediately after hearing your child out, reinforce the separation between listening and deciding by pausing before announcing your resolution.

Even after you learn to delay responding by listening to your child's arguments, you may not be able to defuse the child's upset if you're just going through the motions. Children know when they're being patronized. Instead of just gritting your teeth when your child argues, try to develop genuine curiosity about what the child is feeling.

> "*Why* is he so adamant about not wanting to go to soccer practice?"
>
> "*Why* does she think it's okay to go to a party on a school night?"
>
> "*What happened* in school today that left him feeling so grouchy?"

Don't jump to conclusions. Ask questions. Listen with an open mind. Instead of agreeing or disagreeing, urge your child to say more about how she feels, what's bothering her, and what she wants.

If you find yourself getting too defensive to really listen with interest when your child argues, develop a couple of automatic responses, such as the following:

> "Tell me all about it."
>
> "Tell me more."
>
> "What do you wish you could do?"
>
> "I really do want to hear how you feel about this."
>
> "Let's discuss it."
>
> "Let's hear what you have to say."
>
> "I'd be interested in your point of view."
>
> "This seems important to you."

You'll find that making a sincere effort to understand where your child is coming from will go a long way toward defusing the emotionality of the situation.

Here's another example from a friend.

> "Lisa [my five-year-old] thought this was the day we were going to go to the Folk Arts Street Festival. When I told her that it was tomorrow, I could tell that we were revving up for a doozie of an

argument. Then I remembered the concept of listening for the feelings, not arguing, and delaying the decision.

"I took a deep breath and knelt down so that we had eye contact. 'You were really counting on going today, weren't you? I know how disappointed you must be.'

"Lisa's eyes well up, and she said, 'Yessss.' She was sure that today was the day we were going. She cried a little, and I just held her.

"When we talked about going to the festival tomorrow, Lisa, who now seemed to feel understood, brushed her teeth and we carried on with our day."

The secret of being an effective parent is establishing firm control of children when they're little and then gradually letting go, letting them become their own persons. The first thing to let go of is expecting them not to disagree with your rules and regulations, not to have their own wishes and opinions, not to argue. The child who's not granted the right to argue is a child who's not granted the right to be his or her own person. Allowing children the right to express themselves not only fosters their autonomy, it also enhances the parents' authority. As long as you choose to listen, you're taking charge.

When problems do develop—such as when children demand the right not only to express themselves but also to control the outcome—it's best to think in circles. Instead of trying to figure out who's to blame, figure out what you can do. There's a lot that can go wrong in doing the most difficult job in the world, being a parent. What thinking in circles teaches is that when problems arise it may not be your fault, but it's always your move.

CHAPTER 4

How to Inspire Cooperation in Your Children

What do you say to a child who never has any homework, because he "did it all in study hall" or because "the teacher didn't assign any"? What do you do with a child who promises to take out the garbage but then never gets around to it? How do you respond to a teenager whose sighs and exasperated rolling of the eyes make you feel about three feet tall? What do you say to the child who disputes everything you say? Has an answer for everything? Never wants to do what's asked?

What parent, having been subjected to a steady stream of "I don't want to!"s, "Do I have to?"s, and "That's stupid!"s, hasn't longed for just the right words to put an end to all that whining and complaining? I, for one, treasure those times when I came up with the perfect rejoinder—just the right response to cut through all that arguing and get my point across—often less than twenty-four hours after the actual argument had taken place.

How to Win Arguments with Your Children

Sean reached for his mother's hand as they started across the street to Dunkin' Donuts, where they were meeting Nancy's friend, Sharon.

"Mo-om, *please!*" Sean whined. "It's *my* birthday, why can't I have what *I* want?"

What he wanted was a set of World Wrestling Federation action figures, including such charming characters as "The Undertaker," "The Rock," and one named "The Godfather" who was supposed to be a pimp. Nancy didn't care that the cartoonish violence of professional wrestling had ceased to shock most people. It shocked her. And she wasn't about to let her son bring that kind macho posturing into the house.

"Sean, you know how I feel about professional wrestling. It's stupid. I don't want you watching it, and I'm *not* going to buy you those figures."

"Mom, you're so mean! What's wrong with wrestling? I'm going to be a wrestler when I grow up."

"Sean, those wrestlers only get that big because they take drugs that make their muscles grow. You should have more pride in yourself than to want to be like one of those awful characters."

By this point they'd gotten to Dunkin' Donuts. Once inside they sat down at the table with Sharon, who was sipping a cup of steaming coffee.

"Do you know what this sweet little boy of mine wants for his birthday?" Nancy asked. "Action figures from one of those awful professional wrestling programs."

"Those men are grotesque!" Sharon said. "You should have more respect for yourself, Sean, than to want to have anything to do with those brainless morons."

Sean looked away. Seeing that he felt bad, Nancy softened. "Honey, it's just that I don't want you brainwashed into wanting everything you see on TV. I don't let you watch professional wrestling because it's stupid and it's not real."

Nancy didn't go on. She didn't have to. This was one argument she'd already won.

When you think of winning arguments with your children, what do you think of? Sticking to your guns? Out-talking an insistent child for once? Maybe both. Nancy may have felt that she won the argument about the wrestling action figures because her intentions were firm, she made her points forcefully, and because her son had no answer for her explanations.

What Nancy wanted to get across to Sean was important. Violence and narcissistic posturing are not the ideals most parents want for their children. However, parents who attempt to "win" arguments with their children by out-talking them or criticizing their aspirations don't convince their children of anything. "Winning" an argument by silencing your child only leaves the child feeling resentful.

In order to get beyond mere obedience—giving up their own agenda to do what their parents want—children need to feel that their interests are understood and taken seriously. They need to feel respected.

What does it take to make children want to cooperate? A large part of the answer is listening to them. When a child stubbornly refuses to do what his parents want, they might say that he's being "unreasonable." You can make an unreasonable child do what you want if you're forceful enough, but you can only make him reasonable by listening to and understanding his side of the argument.

Children learn who they are by looking in their parents' eyes and seeing reflections of themselves. Suppose a one-year-old toddles across the floor on shaky legs, then suddenly loses her balance and falls down. She knows it hurts, but she isn't sure how to react; so she looks to her mother for clues. If her mother looks terrified and runs toward her shouting "Oh, my God!" she knows that something awful has happened and bursts into tears. Or, if that same mother, seeing that there was no serious injury, calmly says, "That's okay, honey, you're all right; go get your Snoopy," the little girl knows that everything is all right, so she dusts herself off and goes on her way. Exploring, it turns out, is okay.

When she gets a little older, what will that toddler see in her mother's eyes when she argues with something her mother says? That she's a reasonable person with a legitimate point to make, or that by arguing she's being a stubborn and annoying girl. Maybe the only way for a girl not to be annoying is never to disagree with anyone.

If a child is able to make herself heard and understood, she feels a sense of connection between herself and her parents. It's that connection, that sense of being understood and respected, that creates the possibility of voluntarily deciding to do something that you may not want to do in order to please your parents.

How Responsive Listening Fosters Self-Respect

Nancy was a sensitive mother who stopped arguing with her son as soon as she realized he was feeling bad. The name of that feeling is *shame*. In telling his mother what he wanted for his birthday, Sean was exposing not only his wishes but also his dreams of what it means to be big and strong. That's why children play at being superheroes, whether it be The Incredible Hulk or Wonderwoman or The Rock or Buffy the Vampire Slayer. They're not little and weak. Oh, no! They're big and strong! They can climb up skyscrapers, fly with a cape, see through walls, and beat up bad guys. People respect them.

In criticizing Sean for aspiring to something "stupid," in calling him a "sweet little boy" in front of another grown-up, and in telling him that his wishes showed he didn't have enough pride in himself, Nancy was inadvertently making her son feel ashamed.

Children should not be shamed for asking for what they want.

When we think of parents shaming their children, we're likely to imagine a red-faced grownup berating a sad-faced child by saying something like "How could you be so stupid!" or "You make me sick!" The truth is that such active shaming, however painful to watch, is less common than the everyday skirmishes in which children expose their feelings and are met with disapproval or even disinterest.

Imagine, for example, a little girl who runs to show her father a picture she drew in school. "Daddy, Daddy, look what I made!" The father's response—"Oh, wow, isn't that pretty!" say, or, perhaps, "Can't you see that I'm busy?"—lets the child know not only what her father thinks of her picture, but also what he thinks of her. It doesn't matter that the father who says "Can't you see I'm busy?"

Shame is the painful feeling of rejection that a child feels in response to a failure to receive the appreciation he or she needs from the people who count most, the ones whose good opinion the child craves.

loves his daughter. What parents communicate to their children isn't what they feel inside; it's what they express.

Parents shame their children in arguments when they criticize *them,* as opposed to the point in their argument, and when they fail to listen to and acknowledge the child's side of the issue. Responsive listening lets your child know that you respect him enough to hear what he has to say.

When Nancy criticized Sean for wanting the wrestling figures, what did he feel? To the extent that his mother was thwarting his wishes, he felt frustrated. To the extent that he felt her refusal was unfair, he felt angry. And to the extent that he felt criticized for having such wishes, he also felt bad about himself. The lesson his mother wanted to teach was that being a steroidal muscleman isn't a good ambition, but the boy was also learning that *he* wasn't a good person for having such a wish.

It's normal for children to dream of being superheroes—even if the culturally shaped form of that wish isn't exactly what their parents would wish. Parents must indulge their children's fantasies before they can give them up. Not give them up exactly, but give them time to evolve into more mature and appropriate forms.

In order for Nancy to use responsive listening with her son's wish to get wrestling figures for his birthday, she might want to separate the process of listening to his feelings from the decision of what to do about them. This isn't always as easy as it sounds. Parents tend to respond sympathetically to requests only when they are inclined to grant them. Showing appreciation for what a child wants when you don't want him to have it takes a little practice. Part of what makes this hard to do is that you're all ready to say "but . . ." as though the important thing weren't the dialogue but the decision.

In order to use responsive listening effectively you have to learn to value dialogue with your children. They, too, may be more focused on the outcome than the conversation, but that's partly because they're used to being told yes or no rather than having their parents show a real interest in their ideas and opinions. Notice that I said "show a real interest in." Responsive listening isn't a matter of saying "Yes, but. . . ." "I understand, you think the wrestling figures are cool, but I'm afraid you can't have them." The point is to get the child to talk at length about his feelings.

If Nancy were willing to try responsive listening with Sean, she'd have to be willing to shift from her own perspective to her son's. She'd have to respect him enough to care what he has to say on the subject that interests him. Children don't develop self-respect from their parents telling them what to think and feel but rather from the extent to which their parents demonstrate respect for them, including their wishes, opinions, and feelings.

Here's what a more sympathetic dialogue between Nancy and Sean might look like.

"Mo-om, *please!*" Sean whined. "It's my birthday, why can't I have what *I* want?"

Recognizing that Sean's whining signaled strong feelings, Nancy might have realized that this was an opportune time for responsive listening. "You really like wrestling, don't you?"

Sean's first response to such an opening might simply be to say "Yes." His focus would be on getting what he wanted, not talking about his feelings. Nancy would have to use a little ingenuity to open up the conversation. One way to get children talking is to appeal to their expertise on something they know more about than their parents. Most children jump at the chance to take the role of the expert.

"So which wrestlers are the most famous? Which ones have their own action figures?" Nancy might ask.

"The number one guy is The Rock. He does this really cool way of winking his eye before he's going to beat up the other guy. And my other favorite is Sergeant Slaughter. He wears Army fatigues and he carries an American flag around the ring after he wins. Those are my two favorites."

In trying to be sympathetic to her son's feelings, Nancy might be tempted to say something like "You really like those guys, don't you?" or "I can understand how great it would be to be big and strong like a professional wrestler." Such comments might appeal to very young children, but to older children they may come across as patronizing. The usual formula for conveying empathy—"I understand how you feel"—isn't usually very empathic, and it usually comes across as an attempt to close off a conversation, not open it up. A more empathic comment is often "I don't quite understand how you feel about this; can you say more about it?" Nancy might try respecting her son enough to be both honest about her own feelings *and* open to his.

"Sean, I guess you know that I think professional wrestling is violent and unrealistic. I don't like the idea of encouraging people to fight with each other. What do you think?"

"Oh, gee, Mom, it's not real. It's just pretend. They don't really hurt each other. But those guys *really are* big and strong, and I'm going to be big and strong when I grow up."

"Of course, you'll be big and strong. Are you going to lift weights or do exercises? How do people get to be big and strong?"

Remember that the fundamental principle of responsive listening is to engage your child in a dialogue about his feelings. How hard is it, really, to get a young child talking about his fantasies of what he might want to be when he grows up?

Most parents don't approve of the values embodied in professional wrestling, but on the other hand most children long to be big and strong. A loving parent accepts her child's dreams and shows that she appreciates and accepts them—and him. At some point, Nancy will want to say no to her son, but the no should be confined to what she will or won't buy for him, not applied to his right to his own daydreams.

As a therapist, I've always been impatient with parents who shame their children into submission. For example, I once asked a father to find out why his daughter felt bad about an incident at the dinner table in which, when he insisted that she finish her vegetables, she got up and ran crying into her room, spilling her milk in the process. Instead of finding out what his daughter had been feeling, the father proceeded to give her a lecture about the importance of drinking milk. As the father explained things, oh-so reasonably, his daughter slowly hung her head. When the little girl's chin finally sank all the way down to her chest, I went over and shook the father's hand.

"What's that for?" he wanted to know.

"Congratulations," I said. "You won."
"I didn't think that was the point," he said.
"Oh?" I said.

At the time, I thought of myself as simply making a point, but the truth is I could have found a less sarcastic way to help that father see what he was doing.

It's easy to see how the father of the girl who got upset about being told to finish her vegetables could have used responsive listening. Instead of giving her a lecture, he could have asked her why she got so upset. In other words, he could have suspended his agenda to show a little concern for what she was feeling. Saying "I really upset you at the dinner table, didn't I?" would be a way of showing her that he cared, and it would have allowed her to elaborate or not.

Sometimes it's easier to criticize parents than to understand the frustration that sometimes makes them act like less than paragons of patience.

But let's give this father the benefit of the same treatment I'm suggesting that he could have given his daughter. Why might he have felt the need to lecture his daughter? Maybe he had a good reason to worry about her health. Maybe his mother had osteoporosis, and he didn't want that to happen to his daughter. Who knows? The point is that I, as his therapist, would have been more likely to get through to him if, instead of attacking him with sarcasm, I'd used responsive listening to find out what was on his mind before addressing what was on mine.

Here's how I might have shown a little more understanding.

After the father responded to my request to find out how his daughter felt by giving her a lecture, I might have said, "Let me interrupt for a second. I asked you to find out how your daughter was feeling, and you responded by explaining why you think it's important for her to drink her milk."

Better to be honest about what you don't understand than to make a pretense of being empathic. Whatever you say, the point is to invite the other person to talk. "I'm guessing that you have strong feelings about your daughter's nutrition."

"Yes, I do, as a matter of fact. She's always been a fussy eater, and I don't want her to grow up to be one of those teenagers who thinks she needs to look like a fashion model in order to be popular."

Like most of us, this father related to his child not entirely on the basis of who she is but on some combination of her behavior and his own projections. Whatever the father's feelings were, my intention as a therapist should have been not just to get him to listen to his daughter on this occasion, but to help him *want* to listen to his daughter, to encourage him to make a habit of it. In other words, just like a parent, I wanted him to want to cooperate. Therefore it was important for me to take seriously his reasons for not complying with what I'd asked.

"I agree with you. It is a shame that so many young girls feel that way. But let me make a suggestion. I'm not sure your daughter will understand the importance of what you're trying to tell her until you've given her a chance to talk about her feelings first. Would you be willing to try again, and this time try to find out why she got so upset?"

"Okay, I guess I see what you mean," he said. Then, turning back to his daughter, "Honey, what made you so upset when I asked you to finish your vegetables?"

"I don't remember," she said softly.

But her father persisted. "Did I hurt your feelings?"

At first, she said nothing. But after a moment of silence, in which her father just waited, she said, "Yes." She took her lower lip between her teeth and looked down at the rug, not used to being asked, or answering.

Her father tried again. "Honey, you know that I just want you to grow up to be strong and healthy. But is there something about the way I said to finish your vegetables that you didn't think was fair?"

"Yes," she said, this time with a little more feeling. "I was going to finish everything, but you were so mean. You're always telling me to eat what's on my plate, and you never give me a chance."

Once his child had gone this far in explaining her feelings, her father might simply have apologized for making her feel bad; or, if he still felt he must, he could repeat how important he thought it was for her to eat well. The point isn't so much what he does or doesn't eventually say but that his daughter is only going to feel picked on unless her father takes the time to listen to her feelings. The same is true, of course, about how this father probably felt about my scolding him for not listening.

Recently, I witnessed one of the harshest examples I've ever seen of a parent shaming a child. A mother was arguing in my office with her teenage daughter about leaving clothes on the floor. Then out of the blue, the mother said, "Well you haven't always shown such good judgment, have you . . . ?" Then she brought up the fact that the girl had recently gotten pregnant and had an abortion. The girl, thoroughly humiliated, stopped arguing. I'm sure she forgot what they were arguing about. I know I did.

What makes a parent resort to putting a child down, dismissing her point of view, attacking the child rather than disputing the argument? Provocation. More than a few parents get locked into an adversarial relationship with their children, which may characterize their whole relationship or just an occasional interchange that gets overheated. By its very nature, an adversarial relationship is one in which you feel threatened, one that makes you want to protect yourself by defeating your opponent. Frazzled parents often feel that way toward their argumentative children. Worn down by their kids' incessant complaining and the restless energy that drives it, most parents get to the point where they would just like to win one argument once in a while. But the truth is, you don't win an argument by defeating someone you love.

The Difference Between Obedience and Cooperation

What parent doesn't want well-behaved children? Imagine being able to eat dinner in a restaurant with your little ones, knowing that you can count on them to be reasonably quiet and to eat what they order. Imagine being able to tell your children to do something and have them actually get up and do it. Was it Shakespeare or Sam Spade who said: "Such is the stuff dreams are made of'?

One of the first families I ever treated came to the clinic because their twelve-year-old wouldn't do what he was told. What I discovered was what therapists often find in families of children who don't do what they're told: The parents weren't united in their efforts to discipline the boy. In this case, the father thought the mother was too demanding. He didn't have the courage to say so, but his lack of support got through to his son. Thus, in fighting with his mother, the boy was standing up to her in ways he saw his father as afraid to. As a result, mother and son locked horns while the father stood on the sidelines, silently disapproving.

My first move to involve the father was to have him talk to his son directly about his latest misbehavior. When the father dutifully turned to his son and said, "We aren't happy with what you've been doing," his heart clearly wasn't in it. The "we" didn't fool anyone, least of all his wife, and she didn't hesitate to say so.

She accused him of not backing her up, of not caring, of not being involved. At home, he'd placate her or turn on the TV. Now, in my office, that wasn't possible, and so he spoke up, perhaps for the first time, saying that he thought she worried too much about the boy and expected too much of him.

Accusations were traded, tears were shed, apologies made, and, six weeks later, things were much improved. The father was spending more time with his son and, when he disagreed with his wife about discipline, he said so, and they talked it over. The boy was now doing more of what he was supposed to do. "But," his mother, complained, "he doesn't do things very cheerfully. I want him to *want to* do what he's supposed to do."

I didn't say anything. I was too busy resenting that they hadn't given me a standing ovation for helping them. But now, a mere twenty-two years later, I think I have an answer.

Parents say they want their children to cooperate, but do they really? According to my dictionary, "cooperation" is a noun that means "working together for a common purpose or benefit." The word for doing what you're told is "obedience."

Parents say they want cooperation, but often what they really mean is that they want their children to obey cheerfully. For them to want to cooperate, in the sense of working together, children need to feel a sense of mutuality with their parents. In order to achieve a mutual sense of purpose, parents need to listen responsively to their children's point of view. Children can choose to cooperate, but they will only do so after they feel they've been heard and understood.

Cooperation is a product of mutual respect.

If you assume that your children are basically reasonable human beings who want to do well, and you treat them with the respect they deserve, they are more likely to respect you and want to cooperate. Children learn by example.

How do you show respect for your children? By allowing them to express their feelings, even oppositional feelings. By listening to those feelings and acknowledging that they're true, for your children. Allowing children to have their point of view—allowing them to

Listening to children's opposition acts to release their resistance.

argue—gives them a chance to choose to cooperate, rather than just to mindlessly obey, or disobey.

When I was in the Army, I did what I was told. If the drill sergeant told me to drop down and give him fifty pushups, I did just that. If he told me to get down on my hands and knees and crawl across a field of machine gun fire, I did that too. I did what I was told because I was afraid of the consequences of not doing so. What I did not do was cooperate. I didn't always do my best, and I never volunteered.

Once during a battalion-wide physical fitness contest, my sergeant was counting on me to do well for our company. There were ten events, and I got a perfect score on the first nine. The tenth was the mile run, my specialty. I ran hard for three laps and walked the fourth. What I told my sergeant was that I had a cramp. But the truth was, I didn't like him. He was mean and disrespectful to me, and I had no wish to go out of my way to make him successful.

Most parents want their children not only to obey but also to do so

You can make your children obey by being a drill sergeant, but you can't make them respect you. You can force them to do what you want, but you can't force them to do their best for you. You can't compel cooperation.

with a cooperative spirit. The trouble is, when parents say they want cooperation, most expect their children to be cooperative without the parents having to earn that cooperation.

Cooperation isn't just a quality of the child; it's a product of the parent–child relationship. If you think of your children's "arguing" as negotiating for what they want, it may be easier to see how your response can help to engender a spirit of cooperation, or its opposite.

Parents typically respond to their children's protests and demands in one of three ways: by giving in, by acting like a drill sergeant, or by listening to the child's point of view before deciding what to do.

"All Right, All Right, If You'll Just Be Quiet!"

One way to avoid arguing is to give in. When you're in a hurry, or you're tired and just want some peace and quiet, it's tempting to give in to your child's demands. Just say yes, and he or she will stop pestering. We've all done it. However, if your children sense that you will eventually cave in whenever they make enough of a fuss, they'll learn to use whining as a weapon to get what they want. Children whose parents make a habit of capitulating to their demands, if they are insistent enough, will grow up to be demanding and selfish people.

Everyone knows what happens when you give in to a child who throws a tantrum. The child will learn to throw a tantrum the next

> **Limits should change for a reason, not because your child has worn you down.**

time he doesn't get what he wants. So why do some parents give up and give in to their children's hysterics? Because doing so shuts them up. It's called *reinforcement*.

We usually look for explanations of behavior in the past. What happened previously to cause a certain behavior to take place now?

> Maria doesn't talk to her mother about what's going on at school? Something must have happened at school to make her reticent.

> Bradley insists on eating only his favorite brand of breakfast cereal? Something must have happened when he was younger to make him uncomfortable with change.

A better place to look for explanations for why someone behaves the way he does is in the future: What happens immediately afterwards?

Maria doesn't talk to her mother? Maybe when she does, her mother doesn't listen.

Bradley insists on his favorite cereal? Maybe when he does, his mother goes out and buys it for him.

Whatever gets rewarded (even by attention) is likely to continue. Whatever gets ignored or punished will gradually fade out.

Suppose a five-year-old starts whining at the grocery store when her mother refuses to buy her a candy bar. The mother gets angry and says, "If you think I'm going to buy you that candy bar when you make such a fuss, you're quite mistaken, young lady!" But suppose the little girl keeps begging and pleading until her mother gets exasperated and finally says, "I'm not going to buy you *anything* until you quiet down!" Suppose the daughter shuts up at that point, and the mother buys her a lollipop as a reward for doing what she was told. What's getting reinforced? The daughter's tantrums, obviously. But that's not all.

Behavior is shaped by its consequences.

The mother is also getting reinforced for giving in. She's being rewarded for her behavior—giving in—by the daughter's quieting down. Family therapists call this "reciprocal reinforcement" to emphasize that the development of unhappy interactions is a two-way street.

As an influence on behavior, reinforcement is powerful—how do you think they teach squirrels to ride bicycles?—and it's invidious. Why do you think parents reinforce so much undesirable behavior in their children? Because much of the reinforcement we offer isn't well thought out. How often do parents make a point of catching their children being good? Children learn to get their parents' attention by pestering. Sometimes they get scolded, but sometimes they get rewarded. The best way to eliminate tantrums is to ignore them.

The life-support system for tantrums is an audience.

Another fact about learning is that reinforcement is most powerful when it's intermittent. If a mouse finds a piece of cheese every time it runs through a maze, it will come to expect the cheese. If the cheese stops appearing, the mouse will soon give up. However, if the mouse finds cheese at the end of the maze at some times and not others, it won't give up so easily when the cheese isn't there. Likewise, the child whose parents occasionally but not always give in to his tantrums will be reinforced to keep trying. Even if they don't give in this time, experience shows, they might give in the next time, or maybe the time after that.

The thing for parents to recognize is that children learn to behave in ways that get rewarded. Even though no parent intends to reinforce tantrums, giving in to them—even, or especially, occasionally—increases the likelihood of their occurrence. The best way to eliminate tantrums is to teach your children the difference between asking for what they want (and being willing to take no for an answer) and demanding it. If you want your children to ask for what they want, rather than demand it, reward them for asking.

The relationship between responsive listening and tantrums isn't what some parents might think. Listening to someone does not, despite how we sometimes use this term, mean doing what they want.

Tantrums are a primitive form of negotiation that reduce the options for response to giving in or holding out. Once children work themselves up into an emotional tantrum, there is no reasoning with them. You can try saying something like "You're really upset, aren't you?" but you're unlikely to get anything through to a tantruming child other than that she's going to get her way or not. Responsive listening prevents tantrums from getting started by opening more mature lines of communication.

In the case of tantrums, the child says "I want this," and the parent says "No." After one or more repetitions of this exchange, the child gets upset and starts crying. A parent who uses responsive listening rather than just saying no gives the child a chance to explain herself— and gives the parent a chance to acknowledge what the child is feeling. This child is very unlikely to throw a tantrum, even if her parent finally does say no. Her feelings don't have to explode in an outburst; they've already been expressed and heard.

Sometimes, if you're alert, you can stop a tantrum before it starts. On a recent trip south on I-95 I stopped for lunch at one of those places that serves baked chicken. It was a Sunday morning and the place was hot and crowded. When I finally got my food and sat down, I couldn't help but notice a family with two little girls, one about five, the other about two. The little one was tired and cranky, but no one was paying much attention. The kitchen was really backed up and people were having to wait twenty or thirty minutes before their food came out.

The two-year-old was whining in a singsong, "I want ice cream, I want ice cream, I want ice cream." She was probably more bored than hungry, but she clearly seemed to be getting increasingly frustrated. Finally, her father, looking annoyed, grabbed her by the hand and told her to sit down and be quiet. That was it. She burst out crying. Who would have thought that such a little girl could wail that loud?

It's obvious that this father could have spotted the warning signs of his daughter getting increasingly frustrated. It wouldn't have taken much imagination for him to have scooped her up and said something about what she must be feeling.

"Are you hungry, sweetheart?"

"Yes!"

"Me, too, how about if we play a little game until the food comes?"

The point is that tantrums can often be averted by giving a child a little attention before his or her frustration level starts to boil over.

Children whose parents listen responsively to their feelings before saying yes, no, or maybe are rewarded for asking for what they want because it feels good to be able to express how you feel and have someone listen. In fact, the experience of being truly understood, and having your feelings respected, can be even more powerful than getting what you want.

"Because I Said So, That's Why!"

Some parents believe that children should do what they're told without arguing. I don't disagree. Parents usually know what's best for their children, and they know what they are (and are not) willing to put up with. When it's time to put your three-year-old to bed or send your six-year-old off to school, there's no reason to put up with a big argument about it.

In order to have a healthy sense of security, children need to know that their parents are in charge. Children may challenge their parents' authority—it's called testing the limits—but it's more reassuring for a child to know that his parents are the boss than it is to grow up without a sense of being guided and protected by strong parent figures.

When a parent tells a young child to do something, there is no need for explanations. Whether it's said out loud or not, "because I said so . . ." is all the explanation a three-year-old needs for obeying his mother's instruction not to write on the wall. Those well-intentioned parents who feel the need to explain why their young children should do this or not do that are blurring the lines of authority. The need for an explanation implies the legitimacy of a debate.

Mrs. Nevins was sitting in the living room trying to talk to her friend Sarah, who'd dropped over for coffee, while her four-year-old daughter, Melanie, ran around the room singing "Hickory, dickory, dock."

When Mrs. Nevins told Melanie to go play in the other room, Melanie wanted to know why. When Mrs. Nevins explained that she and Sarah wanted to talk, Melanie said, "But *why* can't I stay?" Mrs. Nevins continued to explain—why she wanted Melanie to play in the other room, why she and Sarah wanted to talk, why Melanie couldn't stay—and after every explanation Melanie continued to ask a series of additional "but *why?*"s.

If you're familiar with this scenario, you know that there are two likely outcomes. Either the mother will eventually get fed up and raise her voice and make threats until the child knows she means business, or the mother will say, "Okay, if you're quiet, you can stay." Neither is a very good solution. The first response teaches the lesson that Mother doesn't mean what she says until she starts yelling. The second response teaches the child that if she whines and then promises to be good, she can get whatever she wants.

If Mrs. Nevins in this example were to be firm and mean business, there would be nothing wrong with her telling her daughter to play in the other room "so that she and Sarah could talk." But this explanation isn't really necessary. What four-year-old doesn't know why she has to play in another room when another grown-up is visiting with her mother?

Here's how Mrs. Nevins could have used responsive listening to cut through the "but why?"'s.

When Mrs. Nevins told Melanie to go play in the other room, Melanie wanted to know why.

Remembering that responsive listening means getting your child to express her feelings, Mrs. Nevins might have said, "What's the matter, sweetheart, don't you want to play in the other room?"

"No, I want to stay here with you."

"I understand. But we're going to talk. So you can either sit quietly over there on the couch or you can go play in the other room."

This brief intervention would probably be enough to eliminate the initial argument. But with a four-year-old it might later be necessary once again to use a combination of sympathizing with the child's feelings and letting her know what her choices are.

When children get a little older, they deserve an explanation when they're asked to do something. Explaining to a five-year-old that we wash our hands before dinner so that we don't put germs in our mouths enables the child to develop the understanding necessary to regulate his own behavior when Mom and Dad aren't around to tell him what to do.

While permissive parents, like Mrs. Nevins, who felt she had to convince her four-year-old to do what she was told, tend to blur the lines of authority in the family, authoritarian parents want their children to do what they're told, when they're told, and without explanation.

Mr. and Mrs. Kelly came to therapy because their previously well-behaved fifteen-year-old son, Anthony, "was becoming rude and disrespectful." Sometimes he'd be out riding his bicycle and not come in the house until fifteen or twenty minutes after he was supposed to. What was worse, sometimes after an argument with his mother, "Anthony would storm into his room and slam the door." My goodness.

Rarely had I met two parents so concerned with what seemed like such minor infractions. What I came to realize was that, in the Kelly family, the transgression in Anthony's behavior was far from minor. At issue in this family was the question of who set the rules.

The Kellys were a close-knit family with four children, Katherine (twenty-two), Mary (twenty), Anthony (fifteen), and Annette (twelve). Mr. and Mrs. Kelly were loving but strict parents. They insisted on neat rooms, clean school uniforms, and, most of all, that their authority not be questioned. Their authoritarian style of parenting worked fine when the children were young. But both of the older two girls had eventually rebelled and were no longer on speaking terms with their parents.

Katherine, her parents told me, was rebellious throughout her teens. She smoked cigarettes, dated boys her parents didn't approve of, and eventually left home after high school and moved to New York. Mary wasn't like her sister. She was a good girl. But, her parents said, it turned out that she was stubborn. She'd met and fallen in love with a boy who went to their church. Mr. and Mrs. Kelly liked this boy very much and were happy for Mary when they became engaged. Mrs. Kelly wanted a June wedding, but Mary wanted the wedding to take place in May. When Mrs. Kelly insisted and Mary refused, it was more than a disagreement over the date of a wedding. Mary's refusal to accept her mother's authority in this matter was a declaration of independence. In the Kelly family, that was treason, and so Mary moved out, married in May, and cut off ties to her family.

May, June, what's the big deal? The big deal is that, once they lay down the law, authoritarian parents expect to be obeyed without argument. To such parents, the idea of responsive listening would seem outrageously disrespectful. Authoritarian bosses don't feel that they have to listen. They make rules, and they expect to be obeyed without discussion.

Your rules needn't be unreasonable, however, for you to be an authoritarian parent.

The Kreegers were a progressive couple who decided to home-school their two children after their second-grader started bringing home various prejudices about minority groups. Mr. Kreeger retired early from his job to stay home and give his children what he considered a better and more liberal education. It turned out that he was a wonderful teacher. By the time the older of the two Kreeger children was in the fourth grade, both children performed better than two years above grade level on standardized tests.

The Kreeger children were also very well behaved. They earned points for doing various chores, and they had points subtracted for misbehavior. Five points for cleaning their rooms, ten points for doing their homework; minus five points for not doing their assigned chores. They lost five points for fighting with each other and *thirty points* for arguing with their parents. In authoritarian households, good children don't argue. Like the proverbial tree that doesn't bend, this rigid kind of discipline often eventually leads to ruptured relationships. Incidentally, one advantage the Kreeger children *didn't* have was contact with their grandparents. Why not? Because the grandparents once made the mistake of criticizing Mr. Kreeger's strict methods of discipline.

Anthony Kelly's mother said something about him that a lot of authoritarian parents eventually complain about: He didn't listen to her. "Listen" in this context meant to obey without question.

There are two problems with authoritarian discipline. The first of these has already been alluded to: Parents can make young children submit without question to their control, but once children reach a certain age, parental authority that doesn't bend will break. By fourteen or sixteen, or twelve or nine, children who don't begin to win some battles will find a way to subvert their parents' authority; and, if they can't find a way to win some battles, they will eventually break away.

The second problem with authoritarian control is that it smothers initiative. You can make children do what you want, and you can refuse to tolerate dissent. But children who are taught to do what they're told without questioning it don't learn to think for themselves.

The hallmark of authoritarian control is insistence on winning every argument. But parents pay a price for trying to "win" every argument. Children whose arguments are never acknowledged as legitimate have only external motivation for doing what they're told. Authoritarian parents rule by coercive control. The last thing authoritarian parents expect to do is listen to their children's complaints.

> **Children should do what they are told because they respect their parents, not because they're afraid of them.**

Children who are forced to do something against their wishes will have little motivation to carry out that decision because they were given no voice in making it. They may comply, out of fear of punishment or disapproval, but they won't cooperate.

Parents who say they constantly have to nag their children to do things are often the ones who think they have an agreement but don't. When an authoritarian parent tells a child to do something and the child who's learned not to argue mumbles "okay," the parent may think the child has agreed. But people who don't get to voice their opinion, people who don't get to disagree or complain often find passive–aggressive ways to express their dissatisfaction.

You can be strict without being bossy. Strict parents set and enforce limits, but if they're not bossy they will understand and accept that their children may not always want to do what they're told. These parents can afford to listen to their children because they know the difference between benign control and domination.

Flexible parents allow their children to complain. What's more, they listen. Sometimes these parents will say, "I understand how you feel, but this is the way it's going to be." Sometimes they'll modify their rules in response to their children's input. You can insist on your authority being respected without failing to respect your children's feelings.

What do children expect from their parents? Love, respect, and appreciation for who they are. Children expect their parents to demonstrate pride in them, not to be too lenient, but also not to be too harsh. Children count on their parents to be on their side, and they expect to be listened to. When children resist cooperating, some part of them is needing or wanting something else. If this unanswered need is not at least acknowledged, the child will not only continue to resist but also feel unrecognized, unworthy, even—at least momentarily—unloved. When children argue, their parents must listen and show some respect for what they're feeling if they want to inspire cooperation.

What can you remember about what your parents did to inspire your cooperation? Did you generally go along with what they wanted you to do? Did they listen to you when you had other ideas? Did they show respect for your opinions? Did you feel safe to argue? Did there come a time when you felt that arguing with them was a waste of time? If so, when did you start sneaking around to do things behind their backs?

Now think about your own parenting. What do you do that helps your children learn to cooperate? Are you aware of the difference be-

You don't have to decide to start modeling behavior for your children; you already are.

tween obedience and cooperation? What do you do to teach your children to think for themselves? What lessons do you model for your children, as opposed to just the things you say?

The Problem of Autonomy

When children argue, it isn't just because they want to get their own way. They are also exploring and fighting for their autonomy, their right to their own opinions and wishes. If parents respond by arguing back, then the child must fight to avoid giving in—not just on the issue at hand but also on the idea that he or she has rights. Children aren't stubborn just for the heck of it.

We want our children to be autonomous—to think for themselves—but we don't want them to be defiant, to automatically oppose whatever their parents and teachers, and later, supervisors and bosses, say. Who teaches children to become defiant? Parents who engage in needless battles for control.

Too much pressure to conform doesn't permit children to grow up to think and act for themselves; it only prepares them for rebelling as the model of resisting pressure. A good example is the defiant adolescent. The defiant adolescent operates in opposition to his parents and other authority figures. His agenda isn't to do what he wants; it's to resist whatever others want him to do. The resistance of the defiant person is based on emotional reactiveness, not reasoned disagreement.

When a two-year-old learns that he can do something at will—like, for example, open the door and run outside, or say "no" to his parents—he wants to do it according to *his* will. In the process of flexing this fledgling self-determination, the two-year-old becomes stubborn, that is, less willing to abandon his own intentions in the face of external pressure. Someday parents will want their sons and daughters to exercise independence—to resist peer pressure to take drugs, to choose not to have sex just because "everybody else is doing it." What's hard for many of those same parents to realize is that in order to develop that kind of self-direction, their children must practice willfulness. One form that a child's willfulness takes is saying no. Another is arguing.

The fate of the child's na-
scent willpower depends on the
parents' response to it. Parents
who misunderstand their children's experience by seeing it
only in relation to themselves
confuse autonomous strivings
with disrespect. To them, a two-
year-old who says "no" isn't

> I once said to the mother of a
> feisty four-year-old, "If you want
> your daughter to think for
> herself, she has to practice,
> doesn't she?" The mother smiled
> and said, "Yes, but can't she
> practice when I'm not around?"

practicing autonomy, he's being disrespectful. (Why are some parents so
uncertain of their authority?)

The child who says no, the child who argues, is learning to find her
own voice. Her parents don't have to take that no as final, nor do they
have to give in to her arguments. But if they deny her the right to resist,
to protest, to complain, they deny her the right to have a voice of her
own.

If, instead of getting defensive, parents accept the two-year-old's
saying no, accept the four-year-old's arguing as a sign of the child's
growing autonomy, the child will learn that she has a right to her opinions, has a right to say what she wants.

PARENT: It's time to come in, honey.

TWO-YEAR-OLD: (*with a big grin*) No!

PARENT: Oh, you want to stay outside and play, don't you?

TWO-YEAR-OLD: (*still singing his favorite song*) No!

PARENT: (*big smile*[1]) Ooh, you're a devilish one, aren't you? Okay,
   in we go, whee!

PARENT: It's time to come in, honey.

FOUR-YEAR-OLD: But you said I could play with the hose, and
   Tommy had it for a long time, and I just got it.

PARENT: Tommy got more time than you, did he?

---

[1]Something as simple as a smile tells your child that you aren't threatened by his resistance.

FOUR-YEAR-OLD: Yes, he always gets more of everything!

PARENT: I know, honey, it's not fair is it? But now it's time to come in. Sorry.

Once a child becomes secure in her ability to say what she wants—and be heard—she can relax her control at will. She can argue, and she can decide to yield. She can disagree with and then choose to go along with her friends, and she can resist and then choose to obey her parents. But the child who is less confident that she has a voice in what happens to her is in a more precarious position. She may feel that she has to refuse to give in to any attempt to direct her. When she argues, it's more serious; she's not just arguing for what she wants, she's fighting for self-determination.

Autonomy and cooperation are not, of course, contradictory. In fact, you have to feel reasonably confident in your ability to protect yourself in order to risk giving in to other people.

Teaching your kids to cooperate by showing them the respect of listening to their point of view has consequences far beyond childhood. When parents are able to listen to their children calmly before deciding on a course of action, the children learn how to listen to the people they encounter in the world. When confronted with someone who isn't ready to cooperate, such children know how to deal with the situation without immediately giving in or demanding that the other person do so.

Responsive listening teaches children to navigate life's obstacles with understanding and greater negotiation skills. When parents listen before reacting, their children will learn to do the same.

CHAPTER 5

Breaking the Cycle of Chronic Arguing

Wise parents establish their authority early, starting when their children are very young, by limiting the number of things they try to control but enforcing essential rules firmly. Having established that they are in charge frees parents to listen to their children's complaints and demands without getting defensive. It's easier to listen when you don't feel your authority threatened.

We've seen how responsive listening can help prevent arguments and instill a spirit of cooperation in children. But what if a parent finds himself or herself already embroiled with a child in the habit of constant arguing? Fortunately, it's never too late to start improving your relationship with your children.

———————————————

As marketing director of a famous amusement park, Sylvia Pratt was considered a tough but fair boss. She set high standards for her staff but was good at delegating and generous in recognizing her subordinates' achievements. Everyone at work respected her. The same was not true, however, at home. By the time she was thirteen, Sylvia's daughter Amanda argued with everything her mother said.

Sylvia wasn't sure that counseling would do any good with such a willful child. She had already consulted a psychiatrist, who put Amanda on Tegretol and Paxil. What she wanted from me, Sylvia said, was advice on dealing with "a disrespectful and demanding child."

As a therapist, I see my job as helping family members learn to get along with each other, rather than as giving advice. Still, if advice was all that Sylvia wanted, I agreed to see what I could come up with.

When I asked her to describe the problems she was having with Amanda, Sylvia made a point of emphasizing that the psychiatrist had diagnosed Amanda as having Oppositional Defiant Disorder. Her stressing this psychiatric diagnosis in front of her daughter struck me as a little defensive. *It's not me; it's her.* But I assumed that such an indictment came from self-condemnation, the universal curse of parenthood.

When I asked Sylvia what specifically she and Amanda argued about, she said "*Everything*—chores, clothes on the floor, dishes in bedrooms—"

"You leave dishes in *your* room!" Amanda blurted out, and just like that they were at each other.

"You leave clothes on the floor all the time!"

"Why don't you ever put *your* clothes away?"

"I told you to put those sheets in the closet!"

"The cats peed on them!"

"You never fold the laundry!"

Who said what? I forget.

When Sylvia and Amanda first sat down and I talked with them one at a time, they were both pleasant and reasonable. But the minute Sylvia began to complain about her, Amanda launched into an argument that had the feeling of a fight that was never finished, only broken off to be resumed later.

When I tried to interrupt to speak to them again separately, both Amanda and her mother responded to me but glared at each other, testimony to the enmeshment that blurs generational boundaries and fuels arguments over not only who does what but who is in charge. Lacking both respect and restraint, Amanda rubbed against her mother's sore spots like a match on a flint, with the inevitable incendiary results.

Clearly this wasn't just an occasional argument. The accusations and counteraccusations that erupted in my office were a sample of an entrenched pattern of arguing between Sylvia and Amanda that characterized their whole relationship, poisoning what was once a loving bond between a mother and her daughter. It took only five minutes to see it. It wasn't just that the arguing broke out so quickly, but that it never got anywhere that made it clear that Sylvia had lost control of her thirteen-year-old daughter.

The Oppositional Child

When parents say their children "argue about everything," it's usually hyperbole. In some families, however, it's true. Some children are so oppositional that their arguing is like a reflex. These children argue not only when they're told to do the dishes or clean their rooms but also about things that don't even concern them, like whether or not it's going to rain tomorrow. It's almost as though they're looking for a fight.

Amanda certainly appeared to fit the definition of an oppositional child. According to her mother, she was "stubborn and insolent." She seemed "to argue for the sake of arguing," regardless of the outcome. I thought it was significant that Amanda felt free to attack her mother in front of a stranger. When challenging her mother, she didn't just make her point or take issue with what her mother said, she tried to demean and discredit her.

In describing Amanda's behavior, Sylvia stressed her daughter's unwillingness to compromise or give in. What struck me was her failure to accept her mother's authority. Amanda behaved as though she were her mother's equal and argued with her as though she were a peer rather than a person of greater authority ("You leave dishes in *your* room!").

Persistent oppositionalism is common enough among children to merit attention as a clinical disorder in the American Psychiatric Association's official diagnostic manual.

> The essential feature of Oppositional Defiant Disorder is a recurrent pattern of negativistic, defiant, disobedient, and hostile behavior toward authority figures that persists for at least 6 months . . . and is characterized by the frequent occurrence of at least four of the following behaviors: losing temper . . . , arguing with adults . . . , actively defying or refusing to comply with the requests or rules of adults . . . , deliberately doing things that will annoy other people . . . , blaming others for his or her own mistakes or misbehavior . . . , being touchy or easily annoyed by others . . . , being angry and resentful . . . , or being spiteful or vindictive. . . .[1]

---

[1] American Psychiatric Association. (1994, p. 91). *Diagnostic and statistical manual of mental disorders* (4th ed.). Washington, DC: Author.

Notice how this description, like any diagnosis, formal or informal, takes the child out of context. *The child* is hostile. *The child* is disobedient. What about the people toward whom the child is hostile? What do they do to trigger that hostility? How do they respond to opposition once it occurs? Why does the child disobey them? Do they set clear limits? Do they enforce those limits with swift and meaningful consequences? What have they done to earn the child's respect?

A child's behavior does not occur in isolation.

Is it really necessary to make this point again? That what children do is related to how their parents respond to them? If you are a parent locked in a pattern of chronic arguing with your child, I'm afraid the answer may be yes.

The longer one is embroiled in a frustrating relationship, the more one dwells on all the awful things the other person does. If you're unhappy with your husband or wife or boss or friend, you probably spend a great deal of time resenting certain things they do and feeling bitter about certain things they don't do.

"Why does he always have to get so angry when I try to talk about my feelings?"

"Why can't he just once show a little interest in my life?"

This focus on the other person, although understandable, is part of what keeps us stuck: stuck in the role of responders, instead of seizing the role of initiators.

There is an additional factor that makes parents trapped in a pattern of arguing see themselves as stuck with a difficult child, see themselves as responding to the child's behavior and not the other way around. That factor is guilt. It's ironic. The myth that says parents are entirely responsible for their children's behavior makes some parents feel so guilty when their children become difficult that they react by projecting blame and denying any of the responsibility they secretly feel.

What I'm suggesting is that, in order to understand a child's behavior, it's useful to look at that behavior in context. What I'm *not* suggesting is shifting blame for children's oppositional behavior to their parents. In families with chronic arguing, parents and children alike feel trapped in the role of victim. After all, what can you do if your children "argue with everything you say"? Likewise, what control do you have over your own life if your parents "won't let you do anything"?

How Chronic Arguing Perpetuates Itself

When arguments in a family become chronic, parents and children stop listening and start reacting to each other. With patience worn thin by pestering and resistance, arguments flare up at the first sign of conflict. It doesn't take much to trigger that here-we-go-again feeling.

In families with a backlog of good will, parents and children are less quick to react defensively to each other. But when every discussion seems to turn into an argument, everyone's fuse is short. Once they become conditioned to expect certain reactions from each other—arguing, not being listened to—parents and children become prisoners of their own expectations.

When arguing and not listening is the rule, children approach their parents with a built-in prejudice. They expect their parents to say no without being willing to hear their ideas. If you assume that your parents don't want to listen to you, then it's only natural to approach them as if concessions of any kind had to be fought for. Thus, children who expect to have trouble being heard tend to start arguing whenever they want something.

In happy homes, parents and children look forward to spending time together; here it's the other way around. Things that should be fun, like a trip to Grandma's or back-to-school shopping, become just another occasion for an argument. Once they become chronic, arguments take on a different character. You expect opposition. You lose patience and sympathy for each other. You aren't willing to listen. Everyone insists on trying to have the last word. Parents see their children as demanding and unreasonable: "They want *everything!*" Children see their parents as unreasonable and demanding: "They won't let me do *anything!*" There's a hopeless, angry quality to arguments that erupt all the time.

When they find themselves constantly arguing with their children, many parents mistakenly conclude that their children are quarrelsome by nature or that they aren't good parents.[2] While understandable, such

---

[2]Those who seem most ready to blame others are guilt-ridden people projecting their own intolerable self-blame.

judgmental thinking attributes too much weight to a notion of fixed personality—and underestimates the extent to which patterns of interaction are fluid, and changeable.

Chronic arguing has a way of reinforcing itself. Parents whose children have a history of arguing come to expect it. The parents' assumption of opposition makes them resentful and impatient, while the children's assumption that their parents are not open to their input makes them confrontational. Over time, these reactions become patterned so that there is a certain inevitability to their repetition.

> Families who get stuck in repetitive patterns, like chronic arguing, often rely on responses to each other that perpetuate the very problems they were supposed to solve. Despite the fact that these measures don't work, they are resorted to time and time again. An examination of these attempted solutions provides clues to family members' network of presuppositions.

Thus, a reciprocal antagonism develops in which children end up fighting their parents, and parents blame their children, instead of learning to be more flexible and tolerant of each other. It isn't just stubborn actions and rebellious reactions that keep families trapped in a cycle of arguing. The behavioral cycle is driven by narrowed perceptions. When children come to see their parents as critical and rejecting, anything the parents do that is consistent with this image is focused on and remembered; anything they do that contradicts this image is ignored or forgotten. Similarly, parents see and remember everything their children do that conforms to the "argumentative" label. These reciprocal controlling images continue to justify their oppositional behavior toward each other, even when this might not be what anyone prefers.

Finally, and most ominously, chronic arguing undermines the healthy structure of authority in a family. A family, like any organization, operates most effectively when the lines of authority are clearly drawn. But when parents and children argue all the time, the hierarchical structure of the parent–child relationship is undermined. Children who argue constantly with their parents lose respect for their authority. They aren't prepared to obey, at least not without a fight, and, consequently, they lose the sense of being under the benign protective control of parents they can look up to and lean on.

Parents whose children argue with them all the time lose the sense that they are in charge and that they are respected. Consequently, they begin to think of their children less as youngsters dependent on their protection and more as antagonists in a struggle for control—in short, less like children and more like adversaries. It is this erosion of the generational boundary (which puts parents in charge and makes children feel protected) that is the most serious consequence of chronic arguing—and the greatest impediment to resolving it.

While an outsider who sees a parent futilely remonstrating with an obstinate youngster might assume that the child's stubbornness is a product of inept parenting, the parent may know that the child has been difficult since infancy. Some children really are hard to deal with. (Some of you are way ahead of me on this.)

Blaming parents for their children's misbehavior is actually a corollary of blaming the child. If a child is bad—disrespectful, oppositional, argumentative—it must be because her parents brought her up that way. Both attributions—it's the child's fault, it's the parents' fault—are based on the habit of linear thinking, according to which relational problems must be someone's fault. The alternative perspective, thinking in terms of circular dynamics, avoids speculation about who is at fault, who started what, who is responsible. According to circular thinking, it's less useful to worry about how problems got started than to see them as reciprocal patterns of interaction, which can be corrected in the present, regardless of what happened in the past.

The question is, once a pattern of persistent arguing develops, how do you break it?

"Why Doesn't She Just Put Her Foot Down!"

When we see a child being rude and disrespectful to a parent, our impulse is to want that parent to crack down on the child. Show that kid who's boss!

Families function best when parents are firmly in charge. The love and understanding that every child needs is more readily available from parents who don't have to fight their children every step of the way. Unfortunately, we live in a time when parental authority is under assault not only from workplace realities that keep parents from spending more time with their children but also from prevailing images in the popular culture.

Television, to pick one very potent influence on the average American child, has made today's children more sophisticated and more cynical. As communications scholar Joshua Meyrowitz[3] argues in *No Sense of Place*, today's children are exposed to the "backstage" of the adult world, to otherwise hidden doubts and conflicts, foolishness and failures of adult types they see on TV. This demystification undermines children's trust and confidence in traditional authority structures. It's hard to maintain an ideal of adult wisdom when your image of a parent figure is Homer Simpson.

Psychologists who encourage parents to reassert their authority over argumentative children recommend setting firmer limits and being more consistent in managing the recalcitrant child's behavior. Good advice. But this get-tough policy works best before a pattern of argumentation becomes entrenched. By the time children are used to challenging their parents' authority, efforts to institute a regime of stricter discipline are likely to fuel an adversarial pattern.

> **One of the frustrations of today's parents is that when they were children they did what they were told. That's what children did. Now they find themselves embroiled in arguments with children who have no such expectations.**

When children become accustomed to lax or inconsistent discipline, any attempt to set firmer limits will lead to power struggles. When parents decide to get tougher, their children's first response is to resist. When power struggles escalate, the parents may eventually win, and they may not, but they will be in for a battle. The worst thing a parent can do is decide to crack down on a child but then give up or back off in the face of increasing resistance. All the more reason to pick your battles carefully.

Sometimes it seems that a parent's only choices with an argumentative child are to get tough or give in. Fortunately, there is another approach.

---

[3]Meyrowitz, J. (1985). *No Sense of Place*. New York: Oxford University Press.

The Two Faces of Parental Authority

The fundamental objective for families with children whose arguing reflects a lack of respect for their parents should be to restore the parents to a position of authority.

When we think of exercising parental authority, we tend to think first of discipline. Parents take charge by setting and enforcing the rules. If the mother of a three-year-old tells the child to go to his room and the child obeys, it's clear who is the parent and who is the child. But there is a second side of parenting, and that's nurture. Parents are also in charge when they act in a supportive, nurturing role with their children. If the mother of a three-year-old sits the child down on her lap and reads him a story, there is again no question about who is the parent and who is the child.

There are two sides to parental authority: discipline (the hard side) and nurture (the soft side). A mother or father who ministers to a child or listens to his complaints is acting every bit as in charge as the mother or father who punishes the child.

> **Parenting is about nurture and control. Whenever parents take the initiative to do either, they are taking charge.**

The essential element in parental authority isn't necessarily making the child do something, but acting in a way to control the nature of the relationship. Sometimes, when children have become chronically argumentative or otherwise hard to control, the most effective way to begin restoring parental authority is to work first on the soft side of parenting.

A Strategic Approach to Reinforcing Parental Authority

The strategic approach to reinforcing parental authority is to avoid power struggles as much as possible and, instead, to look for opportunities to initiate nurturing interactions. Note the emphasis on *initiating*. Argumentative children undermine the hierarchy in a family because their arguments tend to set the tone, a climate in which they challenge whatever their parents tell them to do, and the parents are reduced to fighting back to defend their authority. One way to circumvent these destructive interactions is to beat the child to the punch by initiating positive interactions on the parents' own terms.

Imagine a mother of three obstreperous youngsters who constantly have to be told not to climb on the furniture, not to bang on the kitchen counter with pots and pans, not to use their toys as guided missiles—you get the idea. The more she scolds them not to do this and that, the more they ignore her, until, finally, she loses her temper and shrieks at them.

The mother's complaint is that her children "don't listen"—meaning pay attention to what she tells them to do. An outsider might advise her to "make them listen"—meaning insist that they obey, and punish them if they don't. This direct approach might work if the mother acted soon enough and forcefully enough; but by the time things have gotten out of hand, this get-tough strategy isn't likely to work very well.

Notice how this mother is trapped in a reactive role. The children set the tone of their encounters with their mother by misbehaving, while the mother is reduced to playing catch up. The strategic alternative would be for the mother to take the initiative, to set a positive tone by approaching the children *before* they have a chance to initiate a quarrelsome interaction. (In some families, parents will have to move fast.)

Instead of scolding her children after they start misbehaving, the mother would initiate some positive, fun activities with them before they start to misbehave. She could take them to the playground (a great place to give kids the room they need to run around), go for a walk with them, give them some chalk to draw on the sidewalk.

This example of the strategic approach to reinforcing parental authority shows a behavioral solution to a behavioral problem. The same strategy can be used to initiate positive conversations instead of waiting to react to arguments.

Suppose the father of a fourteen-year-old boy finds that most of his conversations with him turn into arguments. The boy usually approaches his father only when he wants something and, when the boy's requests aren't reasonable, the father has to say no, at which point an argument ensues. Meanwhile the father tries to avoid hassling his son and only brings up things like the dirty dishes in the living room after he gets really fed up. Once again, an argument ensues. Thus, father and son are caught in a cycle of arguing, one result of which is that the boy stops treating his father with respect.

Here the father could attempt to break the pattern of arguing and disrespect by looking for opportunities to initiate positive conversations on subjects his son might enjoy. With a fourteen-year-old, this may take a little ingenuity. Teenagers often don't expect their parents to listen to them, at least not without becoming critical. Some possibilities would be to ask the son for information on some subject he prides himself on knowing something about—sports, cars, the son's hobbies, neutral discussions about third parties—in other words, anything that's not likely to be contentious and isn't too intrusive.

The strategy of parents reinforcing their children's respect by initiating positive activities and conversations isn't designed to be an all-purpose solution to family problems. Rather it is designed as the opening wedge in a strategy to break down the expectation that every conversation will end in an argument.

Because listening and parental authority go hand in hand, learning to listen helps put you in charge.

Responsive listening plays a key role in working on the soft side of parental authority, because the parent who is getting a child to open up is in control of the interaction.

Remember that listening to what your children want isn't the same as letting them *do* whatever they want. Unless you doubt your authority, "winning" an argument with someone you love means that both sides emerge with a sense of having been heard and understood.

The shift from arguing with a child's protests to hearing him out—even drawing him out—is a shift from being defensive to taking charge, and it transforms the whole nature of the relationship. Instead of seeing their parents as antagonists, listened-to children begin to think of them as people interested in hearing what they have to say, people who understand, people who care. Will they automatically give up their wish to stay up past bedtime or immediately start putting away all their dirty dishes? No, but the child who feels understood is more likely to cooperate, especially when it becomes clear that the parents' decision-making authority is not open to discussion.

When parents start listening, really listening, without lecturing or criticizing, children gradually start opening up to them. Instead of seeing their parents as jailers or critics, listened-to children are willing to talk about their experience because they know that their feelings will be respected. By listening, parents start learning more about what's going on in their children's lives, what they think, why they feel the way they do. Issues of control don't cease to exist, but when the basic tenor of the relationship is changed from arguing to understanding, children become more accepting of their parents' authority.

One of the unfortunate side effects of chronic arguing is that children become angry and bitter. They expect conversations to be adversarial, so they close themselves off from their parents for self-protection.

"How was school today?"

"Fine."

When conversations take on this brief, perfunctory nature, more and more of the child's world of experience is sealed off from his parents. Children talk to their friends, of course, because they expect to be listened to.[4] Once parents begin to establish that they, too, are friends, by listening responsively, without always criticizing or giving advice, their children will gradually begin to open up more to them.

One thing you can count on: everybody likes to be listened to. Even the most uncommunicative husband or reticent child likes to talk and be listened to. The trick is to establish that you are a good listener. This may take time, and persistence. Nothing changes overnight. Meanwhile, it's important to recognize that even when parents are ready to make a heroic effort to reverse a pattern of chronic arguing, their children may take some convincing.

In order to seize the advantage that listening offers mothers and fathers in strategically reinforcing their parental authority, it's important to look for opportunities to initiate positive interactions rather than just

---

[4]One reason some children have few friends is that they've been hurt so much by not being listened to that they withdraw to protect themselves.

waiting for the chance to be a good listener. Seeking out opportunities to draw your children out and listen to them is one but only one way to create positive hierarchical encounters. Listening is a means to an end, and the end is creating interactions in which the parent is in charge.

Tom and Gina Robards came to therapy because they were exasperated with their fourteen-year-old daughter, Danielle. According to her mother, "Danielle lies, gets in trouble, has poor grades in school, and argues with everything we say."

"She argues with everything you say?" I repeated. "Why do you think that is?"

"The arguing has been going on as long as we can remember," Gina answered. "Ever since she was little, she argues about everything."

Tom agreed. "We thought we could deal with it ourselves, but it's just gotten worse. We've tried everything, but nothing works. That's why we're here."

Like many parents who find themselves caught up in a pattern of contentious arguments with their children, the Robardses mistakenly concluded that their daughter was bad ("negativistic," "rebellious," "defiant"). Underneath that was the fear that they just weren't good parents.

Tom and Gina's previous attempts to control Danielle's lying and arguing only led to painful escalations of the kind of arguments that created this pattern in the first place. The alternative strategy I suggested was to avoid power struggles and instead reinforce their parental authority by initiating positive conversations with Danielle in which they as parents controlled the tone by listening responsively.

"The point," I said, "isn't to placate, but to reestablish your authority strategically. This means avoiding as many fights as possible, letting go of inessential issues, and postponing dealing with essential ones until you as parents can set the mood."

"What do you mean by 'letting things go'?" Tom wanted to know. "Are we supposed to let Danielle do whatever she wants?"

"No," I said, "but are there any relatively minor issues that you regularly have to get after Danielle about that you'd be willing to ignore for a week?"

Gina suggested that they could stop getting after Danielle for leaving her clothes on the floor for a week.

"Why shouldn't a fourteen-year-old be expected to put her clothes away just like anyone else?" Tom demanded.

"I completely agree with you," I said. "In fact, I hate it when kids leave their things all over the house. But what I'm trying to suggest is an experiment, for one week, to see if doing whatever you can to avoid fights with Danielle and trying to initiate positive conversations can help break this pattern of chronic arguing."

Gina thought this strategy was worth a try. "Why not? We've tried everything else."

Tom wasn't so sure. "We'll see," he said.

The following week, I met with Tom and Gina to get a progress report on their efforts to use responsive listening to cut down on arguing with Danielle.

"I tried to do what you suggested," Gina said, "but even when I did try to listen, Danielle would end up picking a fight with me. Once when she got mad at me for never having anything in the house to eat that she likes, I told her I was sorry, and I asked her what kinds of things she'd like me to buy. That worked out pretty well, but whenever I tried to *start* a conversation, she'd just get annoyed.

"The day after our last appointment, I asked her how things were going at school, and she just got mad and told me to stop bugging her all the time. The same thing happened again yesterday when I tried to ask her about soccer. I just can't talk to her anymore."

There were, it seemed, few safe subjects between Danielle and her parents. When a relationship has become this contentious, seeking opportunities to invite conversation on subjects children want to talk about can be an uphill battle. So, I encouraged Gina and Tom to switch strategies.

Since trying to initiate positive conversations with Danielle hadn't worked out so well, I suggested that they try instead to initiate pleasant activities. When a relationship is conflicted, it can be harder to talk comfortably than to do something fun together. Even though many things are likely to lead to arguments ("That was a stop sign you just went through, young lady!"), there are almost always some activities that are likely to be relatively conflict free. If you can't take your child out to dinner without getting into an argument, maybe you can take her shopping for school clothes. If buying clothes only leads to fights, then perhaps baking cookies together or taking your child and a friend to the movies is a better idea.

The more troubled the relationship, the less intimate the shared activity should be. The point isn't to spend quality time together; the point is for the parents to create a shift in the relationship by initiating positive interactions as a way to begin controlling the mood in the relationship.

What Gina decided to invite Danielle to do was help her pick out some tulips for the front yard. "She seemed to enjoy having a say in what color tulips we bought, and when we got home, she surprised me by volunteering to help me plant the bulbs," Gina reported. "While we were putting in the tulips, I tried again asking her how things were going at school. This time she told me that she was doing okay except that she had had a fight with her friend Bonnie. I was pleased that she opened up enough to tell me that, and I made a point of just listening and not pressing for too many details."

All in all, Gina was optimistic about this new direction in her relationship with Danielle. Tom, however, didn't like the idea of "giving in" and "rewarding" a child who was being so disrespectful to her parents.

Like Tom, a lot of parents balk at the idea of trying to be nice to a quarrelsome kid. They see it as appeasement. This is not an unreasonable concern. This strategy does tend to let kids off the hook, at least in the short run. But sometimes it's necessary to take the long view.

Some of you might be wondering how should one parent, like Gina, respond if the other parent remains resistant to the idea of responsive listening?

She could try responsive listening with her husband. Some parents are afraid to draw their partners out on matters that they disagree on. Once again the fear is that if you hear and acknowledge a difference of opinion, you may have to give in to it. Often the opposite is true. Most people feel better, even where there is a disagreement, if their partner at least shows respect for their point of view.

Gina could ask Tom to explain why he doesn't think responsive listening would be a good strategy to work toward gaining control of

> Sometimes it's easier to rethink an opinion after it's been voiced than when it's held inside, unspoken and unexamined.

Danielle. Doing so might help her enlist his cooperation, even if she were only humoring him. Of course, it would probably be preferable for her to take a sincere interest in her partner's point of view—even if she ended up disagreeing with it. Remember: a discussion can always be separated from a decision.

Parents caught up in a cycle of disrespect typically try to think of ways to deal with arguments when they occur. At that point, especially with highly quarrelsome children, there's not much you can do. What I'm suggesting is to seize the initiative by trying to avoid arguments and concentrate on creating a shift in the way children react to their parents. No, this strategy doesn't force children to be respectful. The hope is that by breaking the cycle of oppositionalism, it will lay the groundwork for creating respect.

> You can't force respect.

Parents who are willing to try this strategic approach for working on the soft side of parental authority might consider the following activities for building rapport.

- Going shopping together for something the child wants.
- Going out to eat at a fun place for supper, just the two of you.
- A special trip together to some outdoor activity—hiking, canoeing, bird watching, swimming, horseback riding.
- Visit a museum you've never been to, but be sure to pick one that will be fun for your child.
- Visit a working dairy farm; take a tour of the city waterworks; go watch the planes taking off and landing at the airport.
- Take a bus ride, or a ferry ride, or go to the end of the commuter train line.
- Turn on the sprinkler and take turns getting soaked; go for a walk in the pouring rain; or put on old sneakers and go for a walk in a creek.

In order to get the most out of these activities, think about how they might provide opportunities for listening to and learning more about your child. Children often start to open up, not when you sit them down for a serious talk, but spontaneously when some enjoyable activity puts them in a good mood. Maybe shopping for clothes together will prompt your child to talk about how she feels about her body or maybe what she'd like to look like. Be careful. These are loaded subjects. Resist the opportunity to criticize. Even if you don't want your ten-year-old trying to look like Britney Spears, be careful to listen responsively to what she wants, how she feels, before offering your opinion. Remember, your ultimate influence on your child's self-respect depends more on your acceptance of her feelings than on any lecture you might give about good taste.

John Romano was worried that his fifteen-year-old son might be taking drugs. He knew that drugs were rampant in his son's school, and he'd noticed Brian spending more and more time in his room with the door closed. Because he wanted to avoid confrontations and denials, John postponed bringing the subject up, hoping he might find a natural opening.

As part of his effort to build a warmer relationship with Brian, John had been trying to take him on some kind of outing once a week on the weekend. As these trips had become more regular, Brian started talking more to his dad. Previously fairly silent around the house, Brian became quite talkative once he and his father were out together. One Sunday in January, the two of them were cross-country skiing in the hills just north of town. Brian talked about school, complained about his sister, and then mentioned that one of his friends had gotten arrested for selling marijuana at the Dairy Queen.

John realized that this was a sensitive subject, so he made a special effort just to listen, rather than to probe or interrogate (as he was dying to do). "Gee, that's too bad," he said.

"Yeah," Brian said, "Tim's a nice kid, but that was stupid, selling pot to someone he didn't even know. I would never do that."

"No?" his dad said.

"No," Brian confirmed. "I've smoked pot a few times, but I would never be dumb enough to sell it."

John was a little upset to hear that his son had smoked pot, but he was relieved that the boy felt he could trust him enough to say so. He wondered if there was more to this story, but he realized that this shift toward Brian's starting to open up to him needed to be protected, and so he resisted the urge to probe further. Now that Brian was beginning to open up to him, he could wait.

In addition to considering how special outings with your child can be an occasion for listening more and getting to know each other, you should think about when and how arguments might come up and how you can minimize them.

When Pauline wanted to take her seventeen-year-old daughter, Kim, shopping for clothes, she remembered what happened the last time they went shopping together. Kim had tried on a pair of pants that were too tight on her and then got mad when Pauline pointed that out.

"Skinny people aren't the only ones who have a right to wear tight clothes," Kim had said.

Pauline shrugged. "What can I tell you?" she said. To which Kim had taken offense and gotten quiet. Then a few minutes later, Kim had tried on a leather skirt, and when Pauline said that it was inappropriate for school, Kim had again gotten mad.

This time Pauline resolved to try to avoid hurt feelings or arguments by not criticizing anything Kim tried on. She wouldn't necessarily buy whatever Kim wanted, but she would try not to criticize her. As it turned out, Kim did try on a couple of outfits that Pauline thought were too provocative, but she stuck to her resolve and didn't criticize. The first outfit Kim ended up rejecting on her own. The second was a skirt and a top that Pauline didn't think was suitable for school. When Kim asked if it was okay to buy these items, Pauline just said, "No, I think we've bought enough things already."

To recap: The usual attempts to control oppositional children often lead to escalations of the kinds of arguments that created this pattern of conflict in the first place. The alternative advocated here is to avoid power struggles and instead reinforce parental authority by initiating positive conversations in which parents control the tone by listening responsively. The point isn't to placate, but to reestablish parental authority strategically.

This means:

- avoiding as many fights as possible,
- letting go of inessential issues, and
- postponing dealing with disciplinary problems until the parent can set the mood.

If instead of waiting for their children to initiate contact with demands and protests, parents seek opportunities to invite conversation on subjects the children want to talk about as well as suggesting pleasant activities, a shift will occur in which instead of fighting with their parents—like equals—the children will feel supported by their parents and hence begin to think of them as adults in charge.

PART II

How to Apply Responsive Listening to Different Age Groups

CHAPTER 6

Young Children

TEARS AND TANTRUMS

For all its famous complications, raising children boils down to two things: nurture and control. Children need love, and they need someone to guide them. These two fundamental principles of parenting, nurture and control, apply from infancy to adolescence, and beyond.

Nurture and control can be elaborated into general guidelines that are applicable to children regardless of age.

Under the heading of nurture comes:

Providing physical comfort
Giving love and affection
Showing appreciation and support
Having respect for children
Accepting children and trying to appreciate their unique qualities

Discipline entails:

Having a consistent approach
Sharing the load if there is more than one parent
Providing clear and reasonable expectations
Setting clear and firm limits
Enforcing those limits

Given the theme of this book, you won't be surprised if I add to these principles of good parenting:

Allowing dissent and expression of feelings
Letting children become progressively more independent as they grow older

Although these principles hold true regardless of the child's age, there are specific guidelines to be emphasized at each stage. Since most parents start to figure out what to do just about the time it's too late, it might be helpful to know a little about child development—but common sense and good judgment go a long way toward filling in the gaps.

Common sense tells us that young children need more nurture than control, and that as they get older, say four or five, control becomes more important. However, here is one of the fundamental paradoxes of parenting: Parents who succeed (or not) in establishing authority and control over their children do so (or not) when the children are very young.

> **By the time they're two, children know whether or not their parents mean business when they give orders.**

Even with very young children, responsive listening helps a parent establish benign but effective control. Instead of fighting with a two-year-old whose answer to everything is *No!* or trying to reason with a toddler who throws temper tantrums, responsive listening teaches parents to distinguish between the child's right to his or her feelings and the parents' right to make decisions.

As early as the day they bring their new baby home from the hospital, listening plays a decisive role in helping parents become attuned to their children's physical needs and learning to recognize their psychological needs and wants. You might think I'm stretching a point to say that listening is important even with infants, but all the elements of responsive listening—tuning in, focusing, being receptive, not jumping to conclusions, not ignoring important signals, not imposing the parents' moods and rhythms on their children—come into play in the earliest months of life.

As we'll see, the effectiveness with which parents learn to listen while nurturing and disciplining their very young children helps minimize arguments later.

Listening to a Baby:
Attunement and Empathy

Driving home from the hospital with a new baby is one of those super-charged experiences that takes only a few minutes but lasts forever. Babies, those smiling miracles of our own creation, are so tiny and cute! Maybe God made babies so adorable in order that everyone would want one, and want to take care of it. In sleep, babies look like little angels, giving no hint of all the effort to come.

The vast majority of a parent's time during the baby's first weeks is spent regulating sleeping and eating cycles. Nature designs things so that parents *have to* listen to their babies. They holler to be fed when they're hungry and wail when they're wet—and somehow they always seem to be one or the other. With a new baby in the house, parents live from minute to minute, always on call.

Listening, in these early days, means paying attention in order to recognize the baby's need to be fed or changed before she gets too upset. Most of a baby's needs are unarguable. Most.

As early as infancy, parents begin to distinguish what they consider their child's legitimate demands. If a baby is crying because she's hungry or wet, attention must be paid. But what if she's been fed and her diaper changed? It's nap time, but she wants to be picked up. Should you pick her up because she's lonely and wants to be held, or should you avoid giving in to her so that she won't get spoiled and expect attention whenever she wants it?

I had my first argument with my darling daughter, Sandy, about seventy-two hours after we brought her home from the hospital. (About two minutes later, I had what was not my first argument with my wife.) It was nap time. Or at least that's what I thought. Baby Sandy didn't think so. She thought it was time to be picked up and held, and, using nature's siren, she made her wishes known. My instinct was to let her cry for a few minutes so that she wouldn't get into the habit of demanding attention every time we put her down for a nap. But how many minutes is "a few"? I thought maybe ten. My wife thought we shouldn't let the baby cry for more than five minutes. Sandy thought the limit should be about two seconds.

On this issue, my wife agreed to do it my way, let the baby cry for a few minutes to see if she'd fall asleep (the baby), which she did. A lot of parental "compromises" work that way. One parent accedes to the other's opinion on an issue that he or she feels strongly about, while on other issues the yielding works the other way around. On this question at least, whether to pick up the baby when she cried at nap time, my wife and I set a pattern of establishing a rule based on our assumptions about what was right for the baby and, of course, what was right for us. Thus, from the very beginning, parents respond not only to the real baby in their arms but also to how they interpret the baby and her needs.

Parents immediately attribute to their infants intentions ("Oh, so you want to see that"), motives ("You're doing that so that I'll hurry up and feed you"), and willfulness ("You threw that away on purpose, didn't you?").[1] These interpretations make it possible for parents to understand their child's wishes, correctly or incorrectly, and to respond, by accommodating or resisting.

For example, a mother who fears aggressiveness might interpret things like the baby's poking a finger in her face, forcefully exploring the mother's body, arm waving, pushing against her, pulling her hair or earrings, and so on as acts of aggression rather than exploration. But maybe the baby became so forceful only when his mother ignored his bids for attention and he was obliged to repeat them at a higher level of intensity to get her to notice. Thus, a circular pattern of misunderstanding is established, a precursor of later arguments: The baby reaches for his mother; she ignores him; he increases the intensity of his efforts to get her attention, which she interprets as aggression; and she responds to protect herself by turning away or putting the baby down. In this scenario, the baby may indeed become more aggressive. Once again, notice that the "argument" here is two-sided, propelled not just by the child but by the interaction between the child's behavior and the parent's response.

Thus, even from the earliest months of life, arguments between parent and child reflect not just opposing wills but also reading and mis-

---

[1]Stern, D. (1985). *The interpersonal world of the infant: A view from psychoanalysis and developmental psychology.* New York: Basic Books.

reading each other's intentions. When an eight-month-old tries to squirm out of his mother's arms, is he rejecting her affection or trying to play? Is he "arguing" or exploring? When an eleven-month-old bangs her cup on the table, is she being naughty or saying that she's hungry? Is she arguing or communicating?

Baby Gerald makes repeated attempts for attention, while his mother, who is stressed and annoyed, refuses to acknowledge his appeals. If it is repeated, this episode will create the expectation in Gerald that to get his mother's attention he may have to become vociferous in expressing his needs. He may have to become "argumentative." Meanwhile, Gerald's mother develops an image of him as always making unreasonable demands.

Misreading a child's intentions is an early prototype of one of parents' greatest contributions to unnecessary arguments with their children—trying to control what doesn't need to be controlled.

When babies are too young to talk, it's up to their parents to understand what they feel but cannot say. Imagine for a moment that you are a baby who hasn't learned to talk and you want something. What do you do if you see what you want but it's out of reach? Simple. You get your mother to read your mind.

Reading a child's mind begins with *attunement*. Attunement, a parent's ability to share the child's affective state, is a pervasive feature of parent–child interactions, and it has profound consequences. It is the forerunner of empathy and the essence of human understanding. Attunement begins with an intuitive response of sharing your baby's mood and showing it.

An eight-month-old boy crawls under the table to get a toy and, as he grasps it, he lets out an exuberant "aah!" and looks at his mother. His mother smiles and claps her hands, sharing her son's pleasure. That's attunement.

When your very own baby looks up at you and smiles and coos, or splashes in the bath, or giggles with delight, how could you *not* love her? Surely, we would like to think, all parents respond intuitively to such communications. Unfortunately, this isn't so. Parents have their own agendas, their own concerns, and their own moods. Some parents are so preoccupied, depressed, or otherwise distracted that they ignore their babies. Perhaps more commonly, many parents respond to their babies not as little people with their own natures, but as projections of the parents' wishes and worries.

Every infant has an optimal level of excitement. Activity beyond that level constitutes overstimulation, and the experience is upsetting; below that level, stimulation is boring. Attentive parents recognize the infant's signal of looking away to cut off stimulation or making eye contact to invite more stimulation.

The next time you see an adult interacting with a baby, notice the difference between responding in tune with the child's level of excitement and imposing the adult's mood on the child. It's an argument without words. The child feels one thing—restful, excited, tired—but the parent doesn't get it. Instead of tuning in (listening) to the baby, the parent imposes his or her own mood (argues). If you see a parent with blunted emotions ignoring a bright-eyed baby, you're witnessing the beginning of a sad process by which unresponsive parents wither the enthusiasm of their children.

Having quite enough unwatered flowers at the office, thank you, I wasn't about to have any around my house. I remember tiptoeing into the nursery at eventide, right about the time baby Sandy was dozing—or pretending to. What my masculine intuition told me she really wanted was not to rest but to be hurled violently up to the ceiling and then come crashing toward the floor—like a skydiver without a parachute—only to be plucked from the jaws of death by Daddy. Whee!

Too choked with joy to speak, the little mite showed her pleasure by widening her eyes like saucers while her face turned a lovely shade of blue.[2]

Excessive enthusiasm may be less depressing, but it isn't necessarily more responsive. "Baby love"—we've all seen grown-ups at it—is the fulsome tone of voice, the honeyed words, the endless marveling and exclaiming.[3] When babies are little, it's almost automatic; babies are so animated themselves that they drive up the intensity of our response.

---

[2]Nichols, P. (1995). *The lost art of listening*. New York: Guilford Press.
[3]Trollope, A. (1881). *Barchester Towers*. New York.

But when this adult enthusiasm regularly exceeds the baby's own, the result is a jarring discontinuity.

The baby whose parents tickle and poke and jiggle and shake her when she's not in the mood is as alone with her real self as the baby whose parents ignore her. This imposition of the parents' agenda is, in what R. D. Laing so tellingly called the "politics of experience," the mystification in which the child's reality gets lost.[4] Not being understood and taken seriously as a person in your own right—even at this early age—is the root of aloneness and insecurity. In the words of psychoanalyst Ernest Wolf, "Solitude, psychological solitude, is the mother of anxiety."[5] Arguing is a child's way of fighting back.

> Loving parents share the moods of their infants and show it. It isn't exuberance or any other emotion that conveys appreciation; it's being noticed, understood, and taken seriously.

Learning to speak creates a new type of connection between parent and child. Language increases the child's ability to make herself heard and understood, and it increases the parent's ability to understand. But language is a double-edged sword. Talking helps children clarify what they want—"I wanna cookie"; "Swing me higher!"—and so cuts down on parents' misreading their children's intentions. But talking also enables parents and children to draw out conflict.

"Arguments" with preverbal children don't usually last long. But once children learn to say things like "I want . . ." and "Okay, Mommy" and "No!" many parents think that an argument isn't settled until the child says "Yes" or agrees to let the parent have the last word.

> With preverbal children, parents always have the last word—their actions are the final say. But parents who insist on their children verbalizing obedience give the children the power to prolong arguments.

When children learn to talk, they become little chatterboxes. At first it's cute. One reason little ones prattle on so is that they're delighted with the magic of this wonderful new skill: They can speak their thoughts out loud! Another reason children talk so much is that this

---

[4]Laing, R. D. (1967). *The politics of experience* New York: Pantheon.

[5]Wolf, E. (1980). Developmental line of self-object relations. In A. Goldberg (Ed.), *Advances in self psychology*. New York: International Universities Press.

talking game is usually played by two people. They talk and someone responds. And they keep talking *until* someone responds.

Remember that it isn't just disagreements that fuel arguments; it's failing to acknowledge what the other person is saying. The name for the ability to put words to what your child is trying to say is *empathy*. Empathy means understanding—not just what the other person says, but what they feel. What *they* feel, not what you might feel in a similar situation. Empathy is achieved by open and receptive listening; it is conveyed by putting what you understand into words.

By the time children get to be four or five, parental empathy (or its absence) has molded their personalities in recognizable ways. The securely understood child grows up to expect others to be available and receptive. The listened-to child who becomes ill or injured at school will confidently turn to teachers for support. In contrast, it is particularly at such times that insecure children fail to seek contact. "A boy is disappointed and folds his arms and sulks. A girl bumps her head under a table and crawls off to be by herself. A child is upset on the last day of school; she sits frozen and expressionless on a couch."[6] Such reactions are typical—and don't change much as the unlistened-to child gets older.

Preschoolers with a history of empathic listening are more engaged and more at ease with their peers. They expect interactions to be positive and thus are more eager for them. They make friends more easily and are happier. They are also good listeners. Already by four or five, empathic failure—not abuse or cruelty but simple, everyday lack of understanding—results in a self that is isolated and insecure, vulnerable to rejection and therefore fearful of new people and experience.

A parent's empathy cuts down on a young child's arguing, because it's easier to accept disappointment when at least you feel that you've been understood. At the other pole of parental authority is discipline. Children argue less with parents who are firmly in charge. So it might seem that there are two separate avenues to cutting down on arguing: the empathic approach—acknowledging a child's wishes, or the controlling approach—letting the child know who's in charge. Actually, empathy and control go hand in hand.

---

[6]Sroufe, A. (1989). Relationships, self, and individual adaptation. In A. Sameroff & R. Emde (Eds.), *Relationship disturbances in early childhood* (pp. 88–89). New York: Basic Books.

The Battle for Control

The title of this section is taken from an unlikely source. It comes from psychiatrist Carl Whitaker's description of the first priority in family therapy. The irony is that Whitaker was the most permissive of therapists. He believed that therapy works best by giving patients complete freedom to open up, to discover and accept their deepest feelings in the presence of a supportive listener. In order to be that supportive listener, however, Whitaker insisted that patients accept his authority to set certain basic conditions—like the time and place of meetings and who should attend—which enabled him to feel comfortable enough to accept whatever patients wanted to say and do within those confines.

Listening is a lot easier when you know you're in charge. It's hard to be understanding in a relationship dominated by a struggle for control.

One reason children argue so much with their parents is that the battle for control isn't settled when the children are young. When a parent's authority is open to question, everything is disputable. "Winning" the battle for control, in the sense of establishing respect for parental authority, is achieved by limiting the number of things you try to control but enforcing essential rules firmly.

With their chubby cheeks and infectious grins, toddlers are so cute that parents often hesitate to be firm in setting limits with them. "Oh, don't touch that, honey," said in a gentle voice may not dissuade a young child from reaching for that wonderfully shiny crystal bowl. The trouble is, once parents fail to establish the precedent that their "no"s and "don't"s must be obeyed, children never learn to accept that their parents have the last word. If the battle for control isn't won at an early age, it has to be refought every time a conflict comes up.

As children begin to walk and talk, their capacity for willful self-expression increases. The toddler can now do things himself. But as the toddler's self-sufficiency increases, so do his parents' expectations of him. His mother now begins to require him to pick up his own ball, to feed himself, not to throw his cup, and so on. The second year of life is a time of

When it comes to avoiding arguments, the number one thing for parents to establish is that when they say no, they mean business.

moving away from the permissiveness of infancy toward the expectations of childhood.

The fact that toddlers can now put their wishes and feelings into words means that their parents can now more effectively understand and empathize with what their children want. This wonderful ability to communicate in words does not, however, mean that setting and enforcing limits should become a subject for debate. When you observe parents arguing with small children, you'll see a lot of the same mistakes. Many of these mistakes involve putting too much emphasis on words as the vehicle for setting limits.

1. *The parent doesn't get serious about setting limits until he or she has repeated the message three or four times.*

While Celia and her friend Rachel chatted in Rachel's living room, Celia's three-year-old, Darla, went over to the bookcase and started pulling out books. "Don't do that, honey, okay?" Celia said, and turned back to her conversation with her friend. Meanwhile, little Darla walked over to the other end of the bookcase and started pulling out books from there. "Honey, please don't do that, okay?" Celia said patiently. Darla sat down on the floor for a couple of minutes, and then, bored, resumed pulling books off the shelf. "Stop that!" Celia snapped. She went over and grabbed Darla's hand and led her to a chair and sat her down hard. "I told you not to play with those books, young lady. Now you sit there and be good!"

_____

If it's easy to see Celia's mistake here in not making herself clear until she got upset, that's because I told this story in a way that made it obvious. But what if *you* are the one who's engrossed in conversation with a friend, and your little one is doing something that isn't, after all, so terrible? So what if she pulls a couple of books off the shelf? What's the harm? The harm is that when parents start making prohibitions without making them stick, children learn that it's okay to ignore their parents until they start shouting.

An alternative to saying no all the time to little ones is to treat their wanting to touch everything as exploration. Instead of telling Darla not to touch her friends' books, Celia could have gone over and invited her daughter to look at the books. Maybe touch them with one finger. And then told her firmly that Rachel's books were not for playing with.

2. The parent makes threats that he or she has no intention of following through on.

Two-year-old Jenny has been playing on the swings, but now her mom, who needs to get home to cook dinner, says it's time to go. Jenny starts to whine and refuses to get off the swing. After a fruitless back and forth, the mother says, "If you don't come right now, I'm going to leave you here and never come back!" The child's eyes widen. Could her mother be serious? As Jenny suspects, and events will confirm, no, her mom isn't serious. The trouble with empty threats is that they teach children that they can continue to resist until threats give way to punishment. Thus a pattern is established that arguments will be prolonged and unpleasant—and won't end until the parent resorts to punishment.

3. The parent uses reason and logic to convince the child to accept the parent's rules.

Some parents have trouble setting limits because they believe that their children should understand the reasons for what they are told to do. While this sounds like a good idea, the natural consequences of not brushing their teeth or failing to get to bed on time are too distant for young children to appreciate, no matter how carefully a parent explains it. Perhaps some parents are intent on explaining why their children should do what they're told because they don't want their children to get mad at them for making the children do things. *It's not me making you brush your teeth; it's the inescapable laws of tooth decay.*

All the explanations in the world are no substitute for listening to your child's feelings. She doesn't want a cookie before dinner because she thinks it's good for her. What "reasonable" parents share with authoritarian parents is a tendency to remain stuck in their own point of view. Explaining, like lecturing, tends to shut off children's opportunity to express their feelings and be heard.

> **Parents who insist on explaining their reasons for setting limits are inviting their children to question those reasons.**

4. The parent uses punishments that don't carry much weight.

When his mother told four-year-old Todd to stop teasing his baby sister, he came back with, "She likes it."

"No, she doesn't," said his mother. "Be nice."

Todd ignored his mother and kept taunting his sister.

When the baby finally started to cry, Todd's mother said, "That's it, young man," and she scooped him up and put him on her lap.

Todd's mother frowned sternly as she held her squirming son on her lap. But from the twinkle in the boy's eye, this looked more like a game than a punishment.

What these mistakes in setting limits have in common is that they allow disagreements to turn into power struggles. Although a certain number of power struggles may be inevitable, wise parents avoid them as much as possible—and, when they must pick a fight, they get it over with as quickly as possible.[7] The ground work for recurrent power struggles—of which arguments are a prime example—are laid down early by failing to teach small children the meaning of "no" and "don't."

Three-year-old Courtney and her friend Samantha were playing dolls at Samantha's house. Courtney and her mother had been there for almost two hours.

"Courtney, sweetie, a few more minutes and it's time to go home," Kathleen said.

Courtney shook her head. "No, I don't want to go!"

"Sweetheart, I know you're having fun and it's hard to leave, but it's time to go now." Kathleen walked over to Courtney and extended her hand. "Come on, honey."

"No!" Courtney insisted and stomped over to the other side of the room.

"Courtney, Mommy needs to buy something for supper before Daddy gets home."

---

[7]Neville Chamberlain, unpublished diaries.

"I'm not leaving!" Courtney said with her hands on her hips.

Now Kathleen raised her voice. "Courtney, if you want to do big-girl things like go on play dates, then you have to act like a big girl when it's time to leave."

Courtney still didn't move.

Kathleen took Courtney in her arms and carried her, squirming and crying out to the car.

On the ride home, Kathleen felt bad about the play date ending in tears, and a little embarrassed for this scene to have taken place in front of Samantha's mother. She stopped at a red light and glanced at the back seat. Courtney was fast asleep with her head flopped to the side. She looked so peaceful and innocent, without a trace of the defiance from a few minutes ago. Kathleen felt guilty about having reduced her little angel to tears.

Kathleen felt guilty for making her little girl cry. That's often the way parents feel when they put their foot down. Like most of us, Kathleen wondered what she did wrong. What she did right was teach her daughter that her mother meant what she said.

When they observe parents interacting with their children, infant researchers often see the parents sending mixed messages.[8] They say no, but their tone of voice and facial expression suggest that they're not serious. In contrast, Daniel Stern cites an example of a mother's response when her infant was about to play with an electric wall plug.

> She yelled, "No!" with great vocal tension, flat pitch, great stress, full facial display, and a rush forward. Such behaviors stopped the infant short. It was thus clear that the infant was given occasional opportunities to see a pure array of prohibitives assembled. Most of the time, however, this was far from the case.[9]

The reason for parents to establish control early in their children's lives is so that they will be in the position Carl Whitaker advocates for therapists—sufficiently in control to feel comfortable listening to what-

---

[8]Kagan, J. (1984). *The nature of the child.* New York: Basic Books.
[9]Stern (1985, p. 216).

ever their charges decide they want to talk about. The principle is simple: knowing how to set limits effectively makes it easier to enjoy your children.

An exasperated mother once told me that she couldn't make her little boy do anything. "He doesn't pay any attention to *anything* I tell him," she said.

"Does he run in front of cars?" I asked.

"No . . . ?" she said and waited for me to make my point.

I didn't say anything.

"Oh, I see!" she said.

What she saw was that getting young children to obey is largely a matter of intention. Is what you're telling them important? Are you serious? Do you intend to be obeyed? Are you willing to put up with an argument? In the next chapter, I'll have some suggestions about effective disciplinary techniques. But these are just details. The main point is that if you don't want your children to argue with you, you have to be serious about your own intentions. But being in control is not the same thing as being controlling.

When it comes to children, the ability to set limits is like money in the bank—it's best not to use it too often.

Responsive listening postpones the need to set limits and, by giving children a hearing for their feelings, makes arguing less likely. A parent who is securely in charge (or decides to act that way) can even make a game out of exploring a child's wishes.

"You wish you could stay up and watch TV for another half hour. No, an hour! You wish you could stay up all night! No, you wish you could stay up forever and ever, and never have to go to bed!"

"You really, really wish you could have a dish of ice cream before dinner. You could eat a giant bowl of ice cream—no, ten giant bowls of ice cream! No, you wish you had a whole swimming pool full of ice cream, and you could dive off the diving board and just swim around eating ice cream! Yum, yum, yum, yum!"

Little children love this kind of thing. (Just don't try it too often; even two-year-olds eventually catch on to manipulative parents.) The playful tone implies that the parent-in-charge isn't threatened by her child's wishes.

When I was in college I had a summer job delivering three-hundred pound blocks of ice to restaurants. The man I worked with was nicknamed "Big Ed the Monster." You can guess why. Big Ed was huge, the biggest man I've ever seen, but the "monster" part was ironic, because Ed was very mild mannered. One time Big Ed and I had a run-in with some guy in a parking lot. He cut us off, or we cut him off, and he got really steamed. He stormed out of his car, cursing and screaming and telling us that he was going to kick us in the part of the anatomy you sit on. I reacted by losing my temper and was ready for a fight. Before I could open my door, Big Ed climbed out of the truck. He just stood towering over this guy and laughing in a voice that sounded like the Jolly Green Giant. "Ho, ho, ho!" The guy turned white. Then he jumped back in his car and drove off.

Is the message here that Big Ed was so big and strong that he could easily have beaten that guy up? No. The point is that, unlike me, Ed was secure enough not to become emotionally reactive. Whereas that guy's hostility triggered my own combativeness, Big Ed remained calm, and so there was no fight. You can't have a fight unless two people play.

Back then, I thought I was pretty tough, and I had been all set to fight that guy. But to Big Ed, that man, who apparently also thought he was pretty tough, was just a pipsqueak, not worth getting worked up over. That's how it feels to be sure of yourself.

The following is an example of how a parent who is sure of herself deals with an impatient little one.

Mrs. Darling had just finished a refreshing day as a substitute middle-school teacher in time to pick up her little Lambkin from day care. As it was only 4:30 when they got home, Mrs. Darling had time to put her feet up and while away a pleasant half hour with *The Complete Works of Immanuel Kant*. Unfortunately, after a long afternoon in the sandbox, little Lambkin was a trifle peckish. "I wanna cookie!" he demanded, using the contraction to save time. "Soon, my pet, soon," his mother, knee-deep in the Categorical Imperative, cooed.

Alas, little Lambkin was at that age when hungry boys cannot be put off,[10] and so the wee lad spread-eagled himself on the Karastan and started howling like a banshee.

"COOKEEEEE!!"

As she reached for her belt, Mrs. Darling recalled what she'd read earlier about "responsive listening." Freshly stocked with wisdom and serenity, she crooned, "I know you're hungry, Sweetums, but just now Mummy is reading. It's okay for you to be hungry—and it's okay for Mummy to ignore you. Okay, Lambkin?"

Stunned by his mother's empathic grasp of the inner Lambkin, the outer Lambkin ceased keening abruptly and started keening at a more leisurely pace. "Cookeee. . . ?"

Reassured, Mrs. Darling spoke further. "Yes, yes, my little one, you wish you could have something to eat. No, you wish you could have something to eat two or three times a day!"

That did it. Lambkin was now as tranquil as a kitten on catnip. "Oh, Mummy, I *was* hungwee," he said to remind us how young he was, "but the fact that you understand how I feel is much more important. I wuv you, Mummy!"

Oh the power of responsive listening! And to think, only yesterday Mrs. Darling had been convinced that the best way to put Lambkin into a more docile humor was with four or five strokes of her belt, administered so as to stimulate circulation without actually breaching the skin.

As some of you may have guessed, this account isn't exactly the way it happened. It's more of what's called a "composite" (by authors who make things up) than a real live example. The principles of responsive listening can be laid out all nice and neat, but what happens in real life is that children sometimes do things to make rational responding difficult. Oh, you've noticed?

If your name isn't Mrs. Darling and your little angel isn't called Lambkin, you might find the following scenario a little more familiar.

Four-year-old Victoria was watching *Clifford the Big Red Dog* while her eighteen-month-old twin sisters were playing on the floor. She was

---

[10]Birth to death.

dressed for nursery school. Her mother, Martha, who was cleaning up from breakfast, called in to her, "Victoria, it's almost time to leave." Two minutes later Martha handed Victoria her sneakers. "Here are your shoes, honey, put them on and then we'll go brush your teeth." Martha, having sensed Victoria's ornery mood that morning, was giving her extra time to get ready.

Victoria shook her pigtails from side to side. "I don't want to go to school today! I want to watch *Clifford*."

Martha sighed. Mornings were not her favorite time. "Victoria, honey, you told me yesterday that you loved school. Your friends will miss you if you don't go. And besides, *Clifford* is on again this evening. You can watch it before supper."

Victoria lay face down on the sofa and pulled an afghan over her head. In a muffled voice, she said, "No, I'm not going!"

"Victoria, it's almost 8:15. I still have to get your sisters ready, and we have to leave in *fifteen* minutes."

Victoria's only answer was to flop down on the floor next to her sister Meagan and grab the doll out of her hand. Meagan began to cry in protest.

"Victoria! I'm not in the mood for this today. If you don't put on those sneakers and give that doll back to your sister right now, there will be no play date at Heather's house tomorrow."

Victoria glared at her mother. "You're mean! I want my daddy!"

"Too bad, you're stuck with me. Now stop it and put your shoes on!" Martha, now completely frustrated and way behind schedule, went upstairs to brush her teeth and get her purse.

She returned a couple of minutes later to find that Victoria had taken the pigtails out of her hair. "Victoria!"

"I hate pigtails!"

"Fine, I'll put a clip in your hair." Victoria allowed her mother to fasten her hair with a large, red clip. Fighting to keep the annoyance out of her voice, Martha said, "Let's put your shoes on."

"I hate sneakers! I want my party shoes."

"You know you can't wear party shoes to school," Martha said and picked Victoria up, plopped her on the sofa, and jammed her wiggling feet into the sneakers.

"Ow, you're hurting me!" Victoria began to wail.

Martha carried her in tears to the car and put her in her seat. Then she got the twins and did the same. Once again there had been a morn-

ing battle. Once again Victoria was late for school. And once again both
mother and daughter ended up feeling miserable.

If you are a parent of small children, you know how awful these
skirmishes can leave you feeling. Can you spot the point at which Martha might have tried responsive listening? How about the first time Victoria said "I don't want to go to school today!"

Whenever a child says "I want" or "I don't want" is a good time
for responsive listening. Another clue that this might have been a useful
point for responsive listening is the exclamation point that indicated
that Victoria was in the grip of strong feelings.

Instead of trying to convince her whining child that she *did* want
to go to school ("you told me yesterday that you loved school"),
Martha might have tried mirroring her daughter's feelings. "You
don't feel like going to school today, honey?" Taking five extra minutes to explore her daughters' feelings might have helped Victoria feel
that her mother understood and sympathized. After all, she's not the
only one who sometimes doesn't want to leave the house in the
morning.

"Might have tried," "might have helped"—yes, in the best of
circumstances. But we don't always have the best of circumstances,
do we? We don't always have the time and patience to be perfect
parents. But here is one of the most important things I can tell you
about the value of responsive listening:

**Upsets happen. No matter how patient you try to be,
you can't always prevent scenes with your children. But you
can use responsive listening to talk with your child later
about what happened—to hear how she felt.**

In this instance, Martha could have spoken to Victoria later in the
day, or even, in the unlikely event that both of them calmed down
enough, on the ride to school. She could have said something like,
"Victoria, I'm sorry we had a fight this morning. I guess you must have
been pretty unhappy. Did I make you feel bad?"

While it's true that responsive listening can head off many
arguments, it's important to remember that it's never too late to
open yourself up as an understanding listener to what your child is
feeling.

Whining

What do little children do when they don't get their way? They whine. They whimper, they beg, they plead—and they keep at it until they either get what they want or drive their parents crazy.[11]

Whining is a young child's most powerful form of arguing. The average two-year-old can whine pitifully enough to make you feel like an ogre for denying her that little something she so desperately wants. When you're out in public, a whiny child's whimpering and wailing makes you angry and embarrassed at the same time. You're upset with your child for being so demanding, and you feel humiliated at the thought that everyone within earshot is thinking what you feel—that if your child is crying so piteously, you must be a very bad parent indeed.

According to Webster, "whining" means "to complain in a peevish, self-pitying way." That pretty well sums it up, except that "whining" is only half of a two-part interaction.

Books on parenting describe two possible responses to whining. The first possibility is, of course, giving in. The second is being firm. One thing experts agree on is that giving in to whining doesn't work. Actually, anyone could tell you that—and they'd be dead wrong.

Giving in to whining works very well indeed. Giving in puts an immediate end to the whining (and reinforces the child's use of this form of arguing). What's more, the parent is reinforced for capitulating—by the child's quieting down. Psychologists call this *negative reinforcement*. Positive reinforcement works to increase behavior by following it with a reward. Giving a rat a pellet for pressing a bar and giving a cookie to a whining child are both examples of positive reinforcement. Negative reinforcement works by removing an aversive stimulus. A rat's pressing a bar to turn off a loud noise and a parent's giving in to a whining child to make him quiet down are both examples of negative reinforcement.

By the way, who are these parents who give up and let their children do whatever they want as soon as they start whining? No parents that I know. What usually happens is that parents scold, lecture, and threaten their children for whining—and *then* they give in.

---

[11]Forty-two percent of all women in state mental hospitals in New Jersey are there because of whining children.

Child psychologists recommend that, rather than allowing themselves to be manipulated by their child's whining, parents should avoid reinforcing this annoying behavior. The most effective strategy is to ignore a whining child. No response, no reinforcement. If whining occurs in public, don't scold or argue. Just remove the child from the scene without comment.

The lesson is that whining leads to exclusion. If whining occurs at home, parents are advised to do their best to ignore it. They should just go about their business without lecturing or fussing. Lecturing and fussing constitute the other half of an argument. Ignoring a whining child means not only not engaging in conversation with the child but also not sighing or giving angry looks. These nonverbal signals are also responses, and they fuel whining every bit as much as scolding.

If you want to eliminate whining, ignoring it is good advice. The best way to diminish any form of unwanted behavior is simply to not respond to it. This doesn't work for things like stealing cookies, which lead to their own rewarding consequences, but it does work for behavior that can only be reinforced by some kind of response from other people. So, to eliminate whining, ignore it. But do you really just want to eliminate your child's whining?

Whining becomes manipulative, but it doesn't start out that way. It starts as an expression of the child's feelings. By using responsive listening you can tune in to a whining child's feelings and shift the interaction from a battle to a conversation.

Whining is a request for attention. If you stop and focus on your child—"What are you trying to say, honey?"—the whining will often stop.

> **When your child whines, make sure you're hearing the message, not just reacting to that annoying tone of voice.**

It was 7:30 P.M. and there were Legos, Barbies, books, puzzles, blocks, and dress-up clothes almost covering the floor of the family room. "Melissa, honey, it's time to clean up your toys," her mother said.

"I'm too tired, Mommy," three-year-old Melissa whined.

Peggy was annoyed at her daughter's whining, but she didn't feel threatened by it. After all, who likes to clean up? Peggy put her hand on Melissa's forehead as though to take her temperature. "Oh, no!" she said with mock horror.

Melissa looked at her mother with wide eyes. "What?'

"Maybe you have the ookem schnookem tired sickness."

"What's that?"

"I'd better tell Daddy. He was supposed to take you swimming to-morrow, but I don't want you to get even more tired. Do you think your sister will catch it?"

Melissa, now beginning to catch on herself, said, "You're silly, Mommy. There's no such thing."

"Oh, that's a relief," said Peggy. "Since you don't have ookem schnookem disease, maybe we could have a race to see who puts picks up more toys. Ready, go!"

In ten minutes the room was clean and both Peggy and Melissa were feeling pleased with themselves.

A week later, Melissa was whining all through supper. "I'm not eating these green beans!" she said.

"But you love green beans," her mother insisted.

"Yuck!"

Peggy looked over at Melissa's little brother. "Okay, I guess Tyler will eat them." And then to him, "Okay, Tyler, here come Melissa's green beans." She put one in her mouth and a few on Tyler's high chair tray. "I don't think Melissa knows how to eat green beans. Do you? You're getting to be such a big boy."

"Mommy, look," Melissa said, "I ate all my green beans!" And sure enough she had.

As you may have noticed, Melissa's mother didn't exactly use re-sponsive listening with her whining. Rather she turned her daughter's protests into a game. Notice, by the way, that in the first example Peggy was annoyed and in the second her first response was to argue— "But you love green beans." However, in both cases, Peggy resisted the urge to challenge her daughter's whiny refusals. She let her child feel what she was feeling. And, although she didn't make a point of specifi-cally talking about those feelings, at no point did she attempt to invali-date them.

Children don't whine just to make noise. They always have an agenda. When a child whines, it's because she's not up to expressing herself in a more mature fashion. She's tired. She's frustrated. She's young. The parent who responds punitively—"Stop that noise!"—is inadvertently supplying the other half of an argument. The parent who responds by ignoring a whining child communicates—"I won't listen to you when you're upset." Or, worse, "I won't listen to you until you get *really* upset." The parent who offers responsive listening—"I can see that you're getting upset"—helps the child learn to ask for what she wants and to articulate her wishes without emotionalism or manipulation.

By taking the positive action of talking with a whining child about her feelings, you can separate responding to feelings, which are always legitimate, from getting into a struggle over disruptive behavior. Taking a positive approach to a whining child gives her a chance to talk about her feelings but doesn't, of course, eliminate the possibility that she may start whining again if you end up saying no. At this point, walking away may be better than allowing the whining to escalate into a tantrum.

Tantrums

Whining turns into a tantrum when a child gives up on asking for what he wants and gives in to feelings of frustration. Now, instead of pleading his case, the child starts kicking and screaming.

Some parents confuse an infuriated shame reaction with temper tantrums. A child who feels humiliated—either by his own failure or for being criticized—may become foot-stompingly outraged. He is I-am-wronged! Let the child who feels shamed rage if he needs to, and storm out of the room if he must.

The easiest way to distinguish between a temper tantrum and a shame reaction is to notice when it occurs. If it happens right after the child has been told no, the message is clear. By screaming and crying, the frustrated child is trying to manipulate his parents to give in to his wishes. The child who feels ashamed, on the other hand, wants to be left alone. Like the child who's having a tantrum, he screams and yells, but instead of throwing himself on the floor in front of his parents, he runs into his room to regain his composure. The shamed child wants to hide.

Unfortunately, adults who don't recognize a shame reaction, or can't tolerate a child's upset, often respond in ways that make the situation worse. They demand to know what's wrong—as if a child convulsed with emotion could say.

The shamed child already has a sense of rage and humiliation, as though his view of himself is being trampled on and belittled. As long as the parent keeps badgering the child, the fantastic wrongness of shame is aggravated by the infuriating helplessness of being trapped and interrogated. If the parent persists and blocks the child's exit, the child's outrage swells to hysteria. Every atom of the shamed child's being screams: "*Leave me alone!*"

The last thing you want when you feel like a fool is an audience. That's the difference between a shame reaction and a tantrum. Tantrums need an audience.

What tantrums share with the outbursts of shame is a loss of control. The child who throws a temper tantrum may be trying to get his way, but he's become too emotional to put his feelings into words.

In responding to a child in the throes of a temper tantrum, the principles of responsive listening still apply, but you must take into account the child's loss of control. First and foremost, avoid responding to a child's tantrum with an argument. Don't just repeat the ruling that made the child upset in the first place—"I said no, and I meant it!"—and never tell a child who's having a tantrum to calm down.

When dealing with a child who's having a tantrum, remember that an argument is a tug of war:

"Yes, you will!"

"No, I won't!"

Telling someone who's upset to calm down implies that they have no right to their feelings.

Avoid escalating the argument by not continuing to verbally oppose the child—"I don't care what you do, I'm not going to change my mind!"—and don't tell the child to control himself. Instead, begin by trying to acknowledge what the child is feeling. Since he's probably too upset to put his feelings into words, do it for him.

"Wow, you're really mad, aren't you?"

Notice, by the way, that putting this statement in the form of a question invites the child to agree. That may or may not be a good idea. Inviting someone to agree leaves open the possibility of arguing. A safer alternative is just to reflect what the child seems to be feeling without asking him to agree with you.

"Wow, you're really mad!"

What I'm suggesting here may seem like an exception to the rule of inviting children to elaborate on their feelings with a question. How does saying "Wow, you're really mad!" still qualify as responsive listening?

The essence of responsive listening is *permission giving*. The idea is to give children permission to feel what they feel and to communicate those feelings to their parents. The reason for not asking a child in the throes of a tantrum a question about his feelings is that he's probably too overwrought to explain. Here a reflection of feelings lets the child know that his parent understands—and gives him permission to elaborate or disagree if he wishes.

Incidentally, most accurate reflections of feeling are punctuated with an exclamation point. Try, for example, saying out loud, "Wow, you're really mad." Then say the same thing with an exclamation point. See the difference? Oops, I mean: What a difference!

Reflecting a tantruming child's feelings won't magically make him calm down. What it will do is let the child know that you understand what he's feeling and, more important, it will avoid the usual tug of war of trying to argue with a child who's out of control.

When they get upset, young children may need a physical outlet for their feelings. The trick is not to try to shut off the feelings but to channel them in a way that's easier to tolerate. Give the child a crayon and a sheet of drawing paper and ask her to show you how she feels. "Here, show me how angry you are. Draw me a picture of what you feel."

What doesn't work to help a child release her feelings is sending her outside or to her room to let off steam. It's important that while she's drawing or punching or pounding that you be there watching. That way you can act as a witness, letting her know that even her most upset and angry feelings are understood and accepted.

If a tantruming child gets totally out of control and starts breaking things, you may have to hold her until she finishes discharging her emotions and calms down. Holding a child who's out of control may be difficult at first, but actually it's reassuring to the child to know that her parent is in charge. It may take several minutes, but she will eventually get tired and settle down—as long as she knows that you are in control.

The Terrible Twos

Somewhere around age two, toddlers discover that they can say *no* to their parents. "*No!*" What a wonderful word. Suddenly the child is no longer little and helpless. Oh, no! She's big! She's strong! She can do whatever she wants!

> Mother calls, "Come on, honey, it's time to get ready for bed."
> Two-year-old Tammy puts her pudgy hands on her hips and says: "No!"
> *What's this?* Tammy's mother wondered. *Was her sweet little girl turning into a defiant child?*

When their two-year-old starts saying no eighty-seven times a day, parents must answer for themselves the question "Is my child becoming defiant?"—whether they do so consciously or not. How parents answer this question goes a long way toward determining how argumentative their relationship with their child will turn out.

In the first flush of autonomy, at about two years of age, children learn that they don't automatically have to say yes to their parents. They can assert their own wills. They can say no.

When two-year-olds start saying no, adults often describe them as "willful," "stubborn," "difficult," or "defiant." These are one-sided descriptions, the product of adult prejudice. Most two-year-olds aren't interested in contesting their parents' authority. They just want to do what they want to do. Don't we all?

Wise parents don't confuse autonomy with defiance. Parents who aren't, or don't let themselves be, threatened by their children's growing autonomy won't let a two-year-old's saying no turn into a contest of wills. A child's no leads to an argument only if her mother or father insists on saying yes, or insists on making the child stop saying no. What's wrong with "no"? It's just a word.

> If you allow your children to become rival forces, the relationship becomes dominated by a struggle for control.

Instead of being threatened by their two-year-old's learning to say no, her parents can take pride in her growing autonomy. A two-year-old's saying no isn't an argument. It becomes an argument only if her parents insist on fighting with her about it. Don't let a two-year-old get your goat.

Just as with whining and temper tantrums, using responsive listening with a child going through the terrible twos can turn a battle for control into an opportunity for communication. Nevertheless, even after you let your two-year-old enjoy the verbal victory of saying no and having her feelings recognized, there still remains the issue of getting the child to do what you want.

When it comes to getting little ones to do what you want, give them choices, so that they can enjoy their newfound sense of control over their lives.

"Do you want orange juice or apple juice?"

"Would you like me to help you into your car seat, or do you want to do it yourself?"

"Which hand do you want to hold while we cross the street, my right hand or my left hand?"

Or if your child has been really naughty: "Would you like a blindfold? Cigarette?"

Encourage children's independence by letting them do things for themselves. Arrange things so that they can do so by making your home more child friendly. Keep cups for water on low shelves, put stools near sinks. One family I know put their daughter's books on a floor-level shelf so that even at the age of one she could pick out her own bedtime story. Another set up a bowl of cereal on a child-sized table and put a little plastic pitcher of milk and cup of juice in the refrigerator before bed so their three-year-old son could get his own breakfast if he was ready to eat before they were up in the morning.

Remember, it isn't always necessary to have a heartfelt chat with your child about not wanting to get dressed in the morning. The spirit of responsive listening is to encourage a sympathetic attitude, even about all the reasons your child doesn't want to do what she's told. But there are times when arguing is just stalling, and you don't have to put up with that. Above all, don't argue with your child's protests. If you have time to listen sympathetically, fine. If not, just make it clear what needs to be done. It is not necessary, however, to be stern to be in control. Making a game out of getting ready puts the parent every bit as much in charge as does taking everything *so seriously*. If you have to be firm and insist that your child get dressed and brush her teeth in time to get to day care, you can let her know later that you understand how bad she feels when she has to rush in the morning.

As we've seen, the secret to preventing arguments with preschoolers is to establish firm but benign control when the children are very young. Parents can avoid arguments by listening responsively even when the little ones are petulant and demanding. Remember that it's easier to listen if you don't allow your rules to become a subject for debate.

When it comes to arguing, the "terrible twos" is a pivotal time in a child's life. Parents who let themselves feel threatened by a toddler's saying no make the mistake of turning a developmental milestone into a battle for control. The terrible twos are like rainy days: They're terrible only if you fret and worry and think, "Isn't this awful!"

Responsive listening is a good way for parents to express acceptance of their children's feelings, but more important than any particular parental action is the emotional ambience that characterizes the parent–child relationship. Children can pass through "difficult periods"—like the terrible twos, the oedipal period, and adolescence—joyfully. The joy they experience is due not only to pride in their own developing maturity, but also to the fact that their development elicits a glow of pride from their parents. Owing to this joy and pride, these periods don't turn into struggles; children's assertiveness isn't interpreted as destructive hostility; and they don't have to argue with their parents to fight for their autonomy and self-respect.

Your little Sean or Melanie says no all day long? Good, that self-assertion will come in handy some day.

CHAPTER 7

School-Age Children

"DO I HAVE TO?"

School is a big place when you're five. Scary, too. You could get lost. The teachers could be bossy. Big kids might tease you. Lining up outside the school door, you notice all the other kids. So many! Most of them are bigger than you. They are first-graders now, or second, or even third. Laughing and poking each other, they seem right at home. You watch for clues about how to behave. Most kids do what they're told. They don't get into trouble. Some kids don't do what they're told. They laugh and joke when they're supposed to be quiet. They don't get into much trouble, either.

From ages five to twelve, children spend a lot of time learning the rules. They learn to conform to the expectations of teachers and principals, and lunch room ladies and bus drivers and soccer coaches and Scout leaders and Sunday school teachers—and, of course, their parents. Some kids learn that if you do what you're told, then you're free to play. Other kids resist being housebroken. Some of these children express their rebelliousness by ignoring the rules, others do so by arguing.

For parents of school-age children, the emphasis shifts from nurture to control. You have to make sure your kids get up and get ready for school, do their homework, put their stuff away, do their chores, turn off the TV and the computer, not kill their little brothers and sisters, brush their teeth, and get ready for bed on time. Arguments now become much more common.

As we saw in the previous chapter, the secret of heading off arguments with young children is to make it clear when you mean business. When children get to be school age, they become more articulate and more insistent about what they want and don't want to

> **Arguments from school-age children are natural. At the same time that they're asked to conform to a myriad of adult rules, they're becoming verbal enough to challenge those rules.**

do. The secret of minimizing arguments with children at this age is to separate arguments and discipline into words and actions. Make discipline about setting clear expectations and applying consequences. Think of arguments as communication.

An argument is, by definition, a verbal tug of war.[1] In order to have a tug of war, both sides have to pull against each other. In order to have an argument, both sides have to argue. Using responsive listening as much as possible lets you turn would-be arguments into conversations.

Is It a Discussion or a Quarrel?

Argue is one of several verbs that mean to talk with others in order to reach an agreement, to persuade, or to settle a question of fact. Others include *debate, discuss, reason, dispute, contend,* and *quarrel. Argue,* the most general of these words, can be used in the sense of a reasoned presentation of views or a heated exchange amounting to a quarrel.

> Erin argued her position so effectively that her teacher had to concede that she had a point.

> Rachel argued so vociferously about what time to come home that her father finally told her she couldn't go.

It is this latter sense, arguing as a contentious exchange amounting to a quarrel, that this book is written to address. Notice, by the way, that I chose different contexts for the two examples preceding. In the classroom

---

[1] *The Complete Dictionary of Words Defined to Support Whatever Point I'm Trying to Make,* by Michael P. Nichols.

(some of them, anyway), children are expected to think about issues. They're encouraged to reason, to discuss, even to debate. What happens at home depends on how parents regard their children's challenges.

A. S. Rancer, professor of communication, points out that arguing isn't necessarily a bad thing.[2] Arguing can be a perfectly reasonable process whereby we go about trying to convince others of our position. Professor Rancer distinguishes between *arguing,* which he defines as forcefully advocating one's own position, from what he calls *verbal aggression,* or fighting, in which one person attacks another person rather than just challenging the other person's position.

Unfortunately, some parents respond to their children's challenging their position as though it were an attack. Authoritarian parents expect to be obeyed without question. They don't tolerate challenges. Arguments are interpreted as an affront to their authority. A child who argues for more freedom, for example, may have no intention of challenging his parents' authority. As far as he's concerned, he's just fighting for his independence. However, if parents insist that respecting their authority means being obeyed without question, then the child must disrespect the parent's authority in order to question their ruling. Thus, whether a child's advocating his own position is seen as a legitimate form of self-expression or as an attack depends on how parents interpret arguments.

Being able to argue effectively is a valuable skill for a child, whereas becoming a verbally aggressive person who attacks other people is a handicap. Arguing stimulates a child's curiosity and increases learning because children seek out information about the issues they argue about. Arguing teaches children to deal effectively with other people and to develop persuasiveness.

The child who questions and challenges is infuriating at times, and often keeps at it long beyond making a point. On the other hand, a child who is willing to argue for her point of view has a strong self-image, and is demonstrating behavior that we often admire in adults.

While the distinction between "arguing" as trying to convince and "verbal aggression" as personal attack is important, we need not give up the familiar term "arguing"

[2]Rancer, A. S. (1998). Argumentativeness. In J. C. McCroskey, J. A. Daly, M. A. Martin, & M. J. Beatty (Eds.), *Communication and personality: Trait perspectives.* Cresskill, NJ: Hampton Press.

to describe children's pestering to get their way in order to accept the point that the impact of children's protests has a lot to do with how their parents respond. By accepting their children's protests as a legitimate expression of feelings, parents can turn what otherwise might deteriorate into a battle of wills into a conversation in which the children get to express their opinions while the parents remain in control of the exchange.

Standing up for yourself isn't the same thing as being disrespectful. If you respect your child's right to argue, your child will learn to respect your right to decide. But the child who doesn't get heard or whose arguments aren't accorded any respect will turn from arguing his points to attacking you. Show your children respect by listening to what they have to say—even when it's inconvenient. Teach your children that it's okay to express their feelings, even vehemently, but that it's not okay to do so in an abusive manner.

It's when people can't challenge another person's position with arguments that they tend to redirect their attack to the person. In fact, research evidence suggests that spouses who are unskilled in verbal argument are the ones more likely to resort to physical violence when they have conflicts.[3] The same lack of arguing skill may also predispose young men and women to accept the conventional myth about date rape—namely, that "women say 'no' when they mean 'yes' to avoid being seen as promiscuous."[4] Thus, not only does accepting arguments from their children help parents avoid altercations, doing so also helps children develop the ability to reason and to challenge ideas.

In studying the styles of parents of five- to twelve-year-old children, Bayer and Cegala (1992) found that encouraging a give-and-take was associated with skill in communication, while parents with an authoritarian ("Because I said so!") style who discouraged responses from their children produced higher levels of verbal aggressiveness.[5]

Once again we see that what promotes arguing is responding to children's protests as an attack rather than accepting their right to dis-

---

[3]Infante, D. A., Chandler, T. A., & Rudd, J. E. (1989). Test of an argumentative skill deficiency model of interpersonal violence. *Communication Monographs, 56,* 163–177.

[4]Andonian, K. K., & Droge, D. (1992). *Verbal aggressiveness and sexual violence in dating relationships: An exploratory study of the antecedents of date rape.* Paper presented at the annual meeting of the Speech Communication Association, Chicago.

[5]Bayer, C. L., & Cegala, D. J. (1992). Trait verbal aggressiveness and argumentativeness: Relations with parenting style. *Western Journal of Communication, 56,* 301–310.

sent and to express their feelings. Trying to stop children from complaining is like trying to build a wall of sand to block the incoming tide. (It's more effective to divert the water into a side channel where the water can end up in a peaceful tidal pool.)

To minimize battles with their children, parents must accept not only that children will resist but also that every child has his or her own unique way of responding.

Different Strokes for Different Children

As any parent of more than one child knows, every child is different. Every youngster comes into the world with his or her own personal style and way of reacting to the world. Some children are lethargic. Others are bundles of energy. Some are intense, whereas others are low-key and imperturbable. Some children handle changes and transitions well. Others don't. Some give in easily; others are persistent and stubborn. Parents who fail to take their children's styles into account when giving orders are likely to provoke more arguments than necessary.

I wish I could tell you that there were exactly six expressive styles among children, or maybe eight. Then all you'd have to do is determine which category your child fits into and you'd know just how to respond. If only it were that simple. In fact, every child is unique. Lest that sound like just a cliché, let me add that the whole point of responsive listening is to help you tune in to the unique experience of your child. The best way to appreciate your child's distinctive perspective is to pay attention and listen. Find out what your child has to say and, in the process, you will move toward respecting his or her own distinct personality.

> **Every child is unique and special. As parents our most important job isn't to mold them into who we think they should be. Rather it is to support them in becoming who they are.**

Benjamin Bradley, age six, is an emoter. When he gets hurt or disappointed, he likes to let off steam. His mother understands that and lets him fume. His father, on the other hand, is the logical type. If Benjamin trips over a lamp in the dark and hurts himself, he might complain, "That darn lamp shouldn't have been there!" His father doesn't want Benjamin to blame others for his problems, and so he's likely to point out that Benjamin should have turned the light on. Which approach do you think leads to more arguments?

Spencer Bradley, age seven, is more logical. When he doesn't get his way, he bombards his parents with reasons why he should.

"He's our 'but-boy,' " says his mother, "as in 'but . . . but . . . but. . . .' " *But* she doesn't like it. Mrs. Bradley finds Spencer's habit of picking apart her reasons for telling him to do something annoying, and she gets impatient with his insistence on explanations. Mr. Bradley, on the other hand, is more comfortable engaging in discussions of logic with Spencer, and the two of them tend to argue less.

Most parents find it easier to accept some personality characteristics than others in their children. Paul likes to know the schedule ahead of time so he can anticipate having to go to the store or out to dinner with the family. Paul's mother, who often decides to do things on the spur of the moment, finds this "rigidity" annoying. Paul's father is more sympathetic because he, too, likes to know in advance when there's going to be a change in his routine.

One reason parents are slow to appreciate the unique characteristics of their children is that we often expect our children to be extensions of ourselves. If we're outgoing and sociable, we expect our children to be the same. If we're early risers, we may be impatient with children who are slow to get started in the morning. When children turn out to have different moods and preferences than their parents, the parents may interpret those differences as defiant or stubborn. But learning to understand your child's temperament can help you take certain kinds of resistance less personally.

Sally used to put up an argument whenever she was told to do her homework at the desk in her room, until her mother decided that Sally just needed to be around the family while she worked. "That's who Sally *is*," her mother says.

It takes Casey three times as long to clean up the play room as her father thinks it should. Watching his daughter stop and play with every other toy she finds on the floor used to drive Nathan crazy. Now he forestalls arguments by letting Casey know what's expected and then getting out of the way so she can do it at her own speed. Nathan also learned not to stand in the doorway, to avoid getting exasperated with Casey's slow and deliberate pace.

Asking a child to behave in a way that runs counter to his or her personality style is like asking someone to sign their name with the wrong hand.

When my son was about ten— no, it wasn't me! When Roger (not *my* son) was about ten, his father— ah, Ralph—joined his son and friends in a game of touch football. The way these boys played the game was nothing like the way Ralph remembered playing it when he was their age. Roger and his friends took a very casual attitude toward the game. They ran out of bounds and then back in again, they said they caught the ball even when it had clearly bounced, and they argued frequently about whether or not a tag had taken place. Eventually, Ralph got fed up and said that they weren't playing the game right. Roger got angry at his father and stormed off the field.

The (anonymous) father's mistake in this example was of trying to impose his way of doing things on his son and his friends. Does this example seem a little too obvious? *Of course* a parent shouldn't try to take over his child's games. Well, the father in question lost sight of this very obvious principle because football was important to him—as important as cleanliness, politeness, or promptness might be to other parents. This father preferred structure and was most comfortable playing within a clear set of rules. His son and his friends, on the other hand, felt free to make up their own rules as they went along. The argument that took place between father and son was expressed in terms of the "right way" to do things, but the fundamental issue was nothing more than a difference in styles.

One way to use arguments as a learning experience is to ask yourself, after the fact, if the conflict was really about *what* to do or merely about *how* to do it. Many of the arguments parents get into with their children have as much to with how the children do things as whether or not they get them done. By insisting that their children do things the way *they* do them, parents often clash with their children's natural inclinations and end up in more arguments than necessary.

When it comes to doing things around the house, many children are slower than their parents. We live in hurried times. Parents may need to push their children to keep up with their own hectic pace—but they can spare themselves a lot of arguments by giving slow-starting children as much lead time as possible.

To cut down on arguments by learning to appreciate your child's unique style, try the following exercise:

1. Describe your child's temperament.
2. Describe your own temperament.
3. See if you can reframe your child's "negative" characteristics as positive, or at least as neutral.

1. *Describe your child's temperament.* Alexander Thomas and Stella Chess, who have followed 133 children and their parents since 1956,[6] describe three sets of enduring characteristics that are apparent throughout childhood and into adult life: "easy to handle," "difficult to manage," and "slow to warm up to other people." Notice that these dimensions are qualities of particular concern to parents. Other researchers, who have tried to take a perspective less colored by the preoccupations of the observer, have reduced temperamental differences to two clusters: watchful inhibition versus fearless exploration.[7] These basic differences produce children who are either restrained, watchful, and gentle, or free, energetic, and spontaneous.

Popular psychologists have identified as many as sixteen personality categories based on the Myers–Briggs adaptation of Carl Jung's personality types.[8] While some parents may find such elaborate typologies helpful, others may find it more useful to focus on their own children's uniqueness and learn to appreciate their most salient personal characteristics.

Among the elements of temperament that parents may want to take into account to minimize unnecessary arguments are the following:

- *Adaptability:* Some children like to know what is going to happen and may argue strenuously if they're asked to do something on the spur of the moment; others are willing to go with the flow. Avoid arguments by giving less adaptable children as much advance warning as possible. If

---

[6]Thomas, A., & Chess, S. (1977). *Temperament and development.* New York: Brunner/ Mazel.

[7]Kagan, J. (1984). *The nature of the child.* New York: Basic Books.

[8]For example, Tieger, P., & Barron-Tieger, B. (1997). *Nurture by nature.* Boston: Little, Brown.

they get upset when you have to ask them to do something without warning, apologize for disrupting their plans.

• *Dependent/independent:* Both sides of this dimension have their pluses and minuses. Independent children are self-reliant but may not respond well to direction. They may be more inclined to pursue their own interests than to work together for family goals. Dependent children may rely on their parents for advice, but they are also likely to be affectionate and cooperative. Dependent children—it might be nicer to call them "togetherness-oriented"—fear abandonment. Avoid arguments with dependent children by accepting their preference for affiliation. Independent children fear engulfment. Avoid arguments with independent children by letting them do what you want in their own way. While dependent children may want clear, step-by-step directions, independent children prefer to figure out for themselves how to do things.

• *Emotional sensitivity:* Most children cry when they get hurt, but some children cry more when someone hurts their feelings. Emotionally sensitive children are highly reactive to *what they perceive as* criticism. These children respond better to requests than to complaints. If you must criticize an emotionally sensitive child, make the criticism brief, and be sure to speak privately and gently when you are correcting your child's behavior. Children who turn inward are more likely to feel hurt; less (apparently) sensitive children may be equally susceptible to hurt, but they are more likely to turn outward. Their response to criticism is to attack. The emotionally sensitive child needs to be spoken to softly and given gentle but unambiguous limits. A more outgoing child needs to be spoken to more clearly than gently, in a manner that leaves little room for power struggles.

• *Energy level:* Some children bound out of bed full of energy; others do better when they're allowed to sleep late. Energetic children can wear their parents out, while their less animated counterparts are difficult to get moving. Avoid arguments with energetic children by taking into account their need for activity. If you give them a tedious chore, allow frequent breaks for them to drain off pent-up energy. Avoid arguments with slow-to-get-moving children by giving them advance notice and allowing them plenty of time to complete tasks.

• *Introversion/extroversion:* Introverted children are serious and quiet. They always seem to be doing things or thinking about something. They love to read. Introverted children can tire from too much social activity and need time to retire to their private preoccupations. Don't fight your child's natural shyness by overscheduling her for activities to bring her out of her shell. Introverts don't dislike people but may be more selective than their extroverted counterparts. They may not talk about their feelings unless asked. Introverts prefer one-to-one interactions with selected people, while extroverted children are energized by being around lots of other people. They may, for example, like Sally in the earlier example, prefer to do their homework in the family room rather than in the isolation of their own rooms. Extroverted children tend to be loud, vocal, and sometimes demanding, especially when they are little. They may need people around them to help them get through what might be thought of as solitary tasks like chores.

• *Optimism/pessimism:* Some children take challenges in stride because they expect everything to work out, while others always seem to worry about what could go wrong. Don't make the mistake of criticizing your child for being an optimist or a pessimist. Children, just like you and me, *hate* to have their personalities mocked. Don't tell pessimists not to worry. And for goodness sake, don't call them "worrywarts." Listen to their concerns. You don't have to agree that things might go wrong—but you don't have to argue, either. Children who are sensitive to hurt feelings use pessimism as a protective mechanism to avoid getting their hopes (and other people's expectations) up. On the other hand, if you feel you need to caution your Pollyannaish child about possible problems, be sure that you first give her a chance to say that she's sure things will go just fine. Acknowledge her optimism as a positive—it is, of course—but add your concerns, and own them as such.

• *Persistence:* Once they accept the need to do something, persistent children will keep at it even when the going gets tough. The trick is to get them committed. Persistence tends to go with independence. These children have determination but often strong wills of their own. Children who are more dependent may want to give up when things get difficult. They are prepared to have someone else take over for them. Get to know what it takes to motivate your persistent child, and expect less persistent children to need encouragement and reminders.

• *Pace:* Some children have fast-twitch personalities, while others are more deliberate. Fast-twitch children won't have much trouble keeping up with your own hectic pace. Slow-twitch children need time to get moving. One way to avoid arguments is by giving slower children a slightly earlier-than-necessary deadline. Expect them to be a few minutes late and plan accordingly.

While you may recognize your own children in some of these temperamental dimensions, you can probably think of other characteristics that weren't mentioned. This list isn't meant to be exhaustive. You don't need somebody else's catalogue to understand who your child is. You need to discover—and appreciate—that for yourself.

> **Work with, not against, your child's temperament.**

2. *Describe your own temperament.* What are your own personality characteristics? Do you like to have things scheduled in advance so that you'll know what to expect, or are you a spur-of-the-moment person? Are you independent and expect others to be the same? Do you come from a family in which children were expected to look after their own homework and possessions, or did your parents keep closer tabs on you?

If you have more than one child, you may find that your personality is very much like one of them, and perhaps very different from another one.

In what areas do you and your child regularly clash? Aren't some arguments about how to do things predictable? It may help to think of some of these clashes as due to temperamental differences, rather than because your child is "stubborn," or "slow," or "willful," or "uncooperative." Most children want to cooperate. They just want to cooperate in their own way.

> **Learning to appreciate your child's— and your own—temperament will help you see many of your arguments as due not to your child being wrong or uncooperative but simply to the fact that your way is different from your child's way.**

3. *Reframe your child's "negative" characteristics as positive or neutral.* If all you see is stubbornness, that's how the child will come to see himself, and that's what you'll get from him.

> "Paul is inflexible. He gets annoyed whenever we have to go somewhere."

> "Paul is a planner. He likes advance notice so that he can anticipate."

Try thinking of "shyness" as "caution," or "stubbornness" as "strong-willed" and see what a difference this more accepting attitude has on your relationship with your child.

Everyone has traits that can be regarded as pluses or minuses. One of my graduate students used to drive me crazy because she did everything so . . . slowly . . . and . . . deliberately. She even talked s l o w l y. But this same low-key approach made her a wonderful therapist. No matter how upset or angry family members acted toward each other, this student always remained calm, reasonable, and reassuring. I'm sure that these same traits will make her a wonderful mother.

Some parents take exception to the implication that they should accommodate to their child's natural inclinations.

"What if my child is naturally lazy? Should I let him lie around on the couch and watch TV all day if that's all he wants to do?"

Coming to terms with your child's temperament doesn't mean giving up control. It means accepting that your child has a basic personality, that he has a certain style of doing things—and, that it isn't likely to change much. Learning to accept, and work with, your child's temperament will help you avoid unproductive battles.

The core of self-esteem is self-acceptance, and the root of self-acceptance is parental acceptance. It isn't just love that children need from their parents; it's their understanding and appreciation of the unique qualities of the child. Children whose parents communicate a basic understanding and acceptance of their temperament grow up believing:

"I am basically okay."

"I love my parents because they accept me for who I am."

How to Discipline Without Getting into Arguments

One of the reasons children argue is to test the limits of their parents' resolve. They think that if they protest long enough their parents will eventually give in. They argue because, at least some of the time, it works.

The way to put an end to arguments isn't necessarily to become stricter. On the contrary, autocratic control may produce obedience—

at least when children are young—but it doesn't create respect, and it doesn't foster cooperation. When it comes to discipline, the most effective control is firm but benign.

Strong parents listen to their children's feelings and, when possible, take their wishes into account. Once they've decided what they want done, however, parents should make their expectations clear, and be prepared to back them up with consequences.

Many parents find that it's easier to be firm when they use responsive listening. Instead of having to choose between being nice (lenient) and mean (strict), they can be nice enough to listen to their children's feelings and strict enough to set firm limits.

> **Effective discipline begins with setting clear expectations.**

One reason children argue is that family rules aren't clearly defined.

Let's say that you've told your daughter she has to clean her room on Saturday before going out to play. If you think that cleaning her room includes putting away all the clothes on the floor and making the bed, but she thinks it means shoving her dirty clothes into the closet, you've got an argument coming.

Cut down on arguments by stating your expectations in a clear, strong, and quiet way. *Clear,* so that your child knows what to expect. *Strong,* so that your resolve is unmistakable. And *quiet,* so that your child hears your message, not the frustration and anger that cloud the channels of communication.

- Make your requests very specific.

Not:	*But:*
"Clean up that mess."	"I want your toys picked up from the living room and put away before dinner."
"Get off the telephone."	"I'll give you one more minute on the phone, and then I'm coming in to see that you hang up."
"When are you going to clean up your room?"	"I want your bed made and everything picked up off the floor of your room before you go out to play."

- Vague requests leave more room for arguing.

  "I thought I told you to clean up your room."

  "I did!"

Remember that there are two parties to effective communication. The single most important thing parents can do to get their message across is to start by listening to what their children have to say. Once children have had a chance to say what's on their minds—and have their feelings acknowledged—they become more receptive to hearing what their parents have to say.

No one is ever really ready to hear what you have to say until they're convinced that you've heard and understood what they have to say first.

When your child begins a question with "Can I—?" don't automatically say no. Stop. Listen. Try to understand where your child is coming from. Sometimes, for example, the child isn't trying to stretch the limits; he or she just needs the rules to be clarified. But you don't have to be a pushover, either. The point isn't to be lenient but to make listening to your child a habit. Don't respond immediately. Take a breath. Ask your child why he or she wants to do something. Think about what the child is saying, and what he or she is feeling. Don't be afraid to take your time making a decision.

  "I'm not sure how I feel about that. I need some time to think about it. I'll let you know after supper."

There are so many times when parents of school-age children have to thwart their wishes that the word "no" comes to evoke a reflexive emotional response. Children hear "no" so often that they develop an automatic tendency to dispute it. "Why not?" "You *never* let me . . ." And the ever popular, "You're so mean!"

It's not always necessary to say "no."[9] Fortunately, there are alternatives:

---

[9]In Japanese business meetings, it's common to hear negotiators saying "I will seriously consider that," rather than saying "no." It is considered a sign of respect to always consider another person's proposal.

- Avoid arguments by explaining why your children can't do something, but without saying no.

  "Can I go over to Tyler's to play now?"

- Instead of "No, you can't," just give the facts: "We're having dinner in five minutes."

- Instead of saying no, acknowledge your child's feelings:

  "I don't want to go home now. Can't we stay?"

- Instead of, "No, we have to go home now," accept the child's feelings: "I can see if it were up to you we'd stay for a long, long time" (as you take her by the hand to go). "It's hard to leave when you're having fun."

Here I'm suggesting letting the child know that you do understand what he's likely to be feeling, rather than saying that you don't as a way to invite him to express those feelings on the presumption that you may not have time for a discussion. If you do have time, by all means take it. In that case, you might ask "Why do you want to stay?"

In order to make sure your children understand what you expect, it's a good idea to remind them gently.

When entering the mall, remind Jennifer that she can pick out *one* pair of shoes, and that they have to cost less than fifty dollars.

Even though you mentioned it the night before, remind Josh in the morning that you expect him to show you his homework assignment that evening.

Reminding should not turn into nagging. Reminding becomes nagging when you use an unpleasant tone of voice, when you repeat yourself several times, or when you go on and on about something. Nagging is so annoying that people block out what you're saying. So then you have to say it more, right? It's a vicious circle.

Danny hates his mother's nagging. "Don't leave your dishes in the living room." "Don't forget to clean your room." "Don't go out to play until you've done your homework." *She's always nagging about something.* This he says to himself, and he gets no argument.

Danny's mother hates that she has to repeat everything before Danny pays any attention. "Why do I have to remind him *over and over* again in order to get him to do anything?"

Nagging follows the same pattern as arguing. It's a game in which two players both play their part. In arguments, two people talk at each other, and neither one listens. In nagging, one person talks at the other, and that one doesn't listen—at least not until the nagging has been repeated several times. Nagging at a child creates a negative atmosphere and results in the child tuning the parent out.

Closely related to nagging as a cause of arguments is making too many rules for children to follow. It isn't possible to control every little thing a child does. Parents who try to control too much end up controlling very little.

Johnny's father likes peace and quiet around the house. So whenever he's home and Johnny makes noise, Johnny's dad scolds him. "Don't sing in the living room." "Don't talk so loud." "Don't play loud music in your room." "Don't jump on Daddy when he comes home." *"Don't shout!"* So many don'ts! Eventually, Johnny learns to avoid his father as much as possible and to ignore most of what his father says when he is around.

Nina expects six-year-old Kylie to be polite at all times. At a company picnic, Nina scolds Kylie for a whole series of minor misbehavior. "Don't run across the blanket, Kylie!" "Don't get grass stains on your jeans, Kylie!" "Don't spill that soda on your shirt, Kylie!" "Don't throw the ball near the grown-ups, Kylie!" Kylie ignores most of her mother's scolding and her obstreperous behavior continues to escalate.

Meanwhile, Nina's friend Roxanne watches as her six-year-old, Holly, runs around playing with Kylie. Roxanne can see that Holly is a little rambunctious but, she thinks, *It's a picnic, let the children have their fun.* Roxanne notices but doesn't say anything when Holly runs across the blanket, when she throws her ball too close to the grown-ups, and when she gets a grass stain on her jeans. However, when she notices Holly grabbing a Frisbee away from a younger child, Roxanne goes over and speaks sharply to her. Holly looks down but heeds what her mother says.

Observations of parents who complain that their children never listen to them show that these parents nag their children over the smallest matters.[10] A parent's incessant nagging eventually comes to have about the same impact as elevator music. It's there all the time, so you hardly notice it.

How effectively parents control their children's behavior is directly proportional to how much they try to control. The moral is don't make too many rules, but enforce those you do make.

Don't state a rule unless you intend to enforce it.

When a parent's idea of discipline is scolding children for every little thing they do, the children don't learn to discriminate between what they can and cannot get away with. What they do learn is that there are no consequences for disobeying their parents.

Consequences

Children argue before a decision is made in order to express their feelings and, they hope, change their parents' minds. After they've done something wrong, they'll try to argue their way out of being punished. The same parents who get into battles with their children about what they should do often end up arguing with them about their responsibility after they have misbehaved. Being reprimanded is no fun, but if it happens often enough, children get used to it. After all, it's only talk.

When people talk about giving children consequences for their behavior, they usually mean punishment. But when it comes to discipline, rewarding children for doing something right is far more effective than punishing them after they've done something wrong.

There is no greater motivator than positive reinforcement.

Behavior that is followed by rewarding consequences is more likely to be repeated in the future. Rewards include such things as treats, toys, prizes, money, stars, special outings, and social reinforcers (close attention, a touch, hugs, smiles, words of approval, a glance, a kiss, or praise). The principle of *positive reinforcement* is so simple that people don't always appreciate its profound implications.

Observation reveals that parents inadvertently reinforce much of

[10]Forehand, R., Wells, K., & Sturgis, E. (1978). Predictors of child noncompliant behavior in the home. *Journal of Consulting and Clinical Psychology, 46,* 179.

the behavior they find most troublesome in their children. At first glance it would seem unlikely that people would reinforce behavior they don't like. Why would a parent reinforce arguing? Why would a wife reinforce her husband's lack of involvement with the children? Why would a father reinforce his son's pestering? The answer isn't to be found in some convoluted motive for suffering, but in the simple fact that it's human nature to pay more attention to the things that go wrong than to the things that go right.

Raymond works quietly on his homework while his father attempts to do his annual duty to the IRS. After a few minutes, Raymond slams his book down and says, "This is stupid!" His father looks up and asks Raymond to please be quiet, "Daddy's trying to concentrate." Another few minutes go by, and Raymond says, "I finished my homework!" "Good for you," his father answers without looking up. Raymond goes to his room and comes back with a football. He plops down on the rug and starts spinning the football on its end. After a few spins, the ball rolls over to where Raymond's father is working. Father slams down his tax form and gives Raymond a lecture about not disturbing him when he's trying to work.

What is Raymond apt to learn from this episode? That if he makes enough noise, he'll get his father's attention.

Parents often respond to problem behavior in their children by scolding and lecturing. These reactions may seem like punishment, but they can be reinforcing, because attention—even from an angry parent—is a powerful social reinforcer.[11] The truth of this is reflected in the common-sense advice to "ignore it and it will go away." The problem is that most parents have trouble ignoring annoying behavior. Notice, for example, how certain words get a big reaction. Moreover, even when parents do resolve to ignore minor misbehavior, they usually don't do so consistently. This can make things even worse, because *intermittent reinforcement* is the most resistant to extinction.[12]

---

[11]Skinner, B. F. (1953). *Science and human behavior.* New York: Macmillan.

[12]Ferster, C. B. (1963). Essentials of a science of behavior. In J. I. Nurnberger, C. B. Ferster, & J. P. Brady (Eds.), *An introduction to the science of human behavior.* New York: Appleton–Century–Crofts.

The way to use positive reinforcement effectively is to notice and comment on specific positive behavior and provide logical and natural rewards.

"Kyle, I noticed that you remembered to pick your clothes off the floor. Thanks, I appreciate that!"

Most parents think they already use positive reinforcement; and they do, occasionally. But parents tend to focus more on the negative. There's a reason for this. We expect our children to behave, and we tend to notice more the times they don't.

> **Like responsive listening, positive reinforcement cuts down on arguments by shifting parents out of an adversarial relationship with their children.**

"You didn't put your books away."

"Your room is a mess."

"Why do you have to argue with everything I say?"

Try this little exercise. Get a little notebook and for one week write down every time you make a critical comment about your child. That's all. Just notice. If you have more than one child, keep a separate tally for each one. Make sure you count comments that start out positive but end up negative. "I really appreciate your doing the dishes, but I wish you'd remember to rinse the soap off next time."

> **Instead of noticing only your children's mistakes, try catching them doing things right, and reward them for doing so.**

The positive alternative to picking on the things your children do wrong is to praise them for doing things right. Make these comments as specific as possible.

"I noticed that you . . . Thanks!"

"You certainly did a good job of emptying the dishwasher and putting away all the dishes!"

"You put your books away!"

"Your room looks so neat!"

"You catch more flies with honey than with vinegar." So if you use honey as a reward, be sure your child bathes regularly.

"You're a big help to me!"

"Thank you for listening and not interrupting."

Every child wants approval for who he or she is and what he or she does.

Even if your children haven't done all that you want, rewarding them for the part that they did do works better than criticizing them for the part they didn't do. One of the most effective ways of teaching complex behavior is by *shaping*—rewarding small steps along the way. Use shaping to reinforce your child for starting to do what you want and then for each step along the way. If shaping doesn't work, either the steps were too large or the reinforcers were too weak.

Even if Susie doesn't always hang her clothes in the closet, you can reinforce her doing so with positive payoffs. Instead of focusing on the times she doesn't hang up her clothes, give her a hug and tell her how much you appreciate her thoughtfulness the next time she does hang up her clothes.

Suppose your two sons fight more often than they play nicely together. Even if it doesn't happen very often, the next time you notice them playing cooperatively together, you could interrupt them with the surprise announcement that you're going to give them a treat. "Hey, guys, you've been playing so nicely together that I'm going to take you out to Friendly's for an ice cream treat."

Some experts warn parents not to praise children so often that it becomes meaningless. I wouldn't worry too much about this. (Take another look at your diary of critical comments.)

Here's a second exercise. For the next twenty-four hours note the number of times you use such social reinforcers as thank yous, hugs, or listening attentively. Each time you do, put a mark next to the name of the family member to whom you gave the reinforcer. At the end of the day you will have some idea of just how reinforcing you are and to whom you direct your reinforcement. Many parents are surprised to discover how infrequently they reinforce their children or that one child gets the bulk of their positive attention. It's not difficult to change this, but the first step is noticing it.

Some parents don't like the idea of using rewards for good behavior because it seems like bribery. If you have to bribe your children, you aren't really in charge, are you? If you reward children for doing what they're supposed to do, they'll learn to demand compensation before they agree to do anything, won't they?

A reward is a bonus given after the fact for a job well done. A bribe is an inducement offered beforehand to motivate the child to do what you want. There's nothing wrong with occasionally saying something like "If you come home with a good report from your teacher every night this week, I'll take you to Busch Gardens on Saturday." The danger of using bribes is that they can shift the balance of power from the parent to the child. A reward conveys that you appreciate your child doing what you told him to do. A bribe may suggest that only if the child accepts the terms of the bribe will he agree to what you want him to do.

"First-and-then": Ideally, a reward is the natural consequence of cooperation. If, instead of arguing or delaying, your child does his chores right away, then there will be more time for playing.

> "If you hurry and change into your pajamas right now, I'll have more time to read you a story before lights out."
>
> "When you've finished your homework, you can go out and play." [Note: "When" works better than "if."]
>
> "Thanks for doing such a good job of cleaning your room. Now I think you have room for a gerbil cage. Let's go to the pet store after supper and pick out a couple of gerbils."

The best reward for a child's doing a good job at his own pursuits are natural extensions of being responsible. The child who works hard at soccer practice is rewarded with increasing skill, more playing time, and the appreciation of her coach and teammates. For a child, a sense of competence is one of the two best things in the world.

The best reward for your child doing what you ask is showing how much you appreciate her doing so.

> "Thanks for helping me with the dishes, honey. I really appreciate your being so cooperative."
>
> "It means a lot to me when you do what I ask without arguing. Thank you for being such a sweetheart."

Knowing that their parents appreciate them is the second of those two things that children love best in the world.

Punishment

Punishment works, but there is a price to be paid. Studies have shown that the family member who gives the most social reinforcement receives the most reinforcement and that the person in the family who gives the most punishment receives

Even if you're already familiar with the idea of positive reinforcement, remember that taking the initiative to set a positive tone in interactions with your children is one of the best ways to reinforce your hierarchical position of authority in the family.

the most punishment from other family members.[13] What goes around comes around.

The best way to deal with annoying behavior is to ignore it, if possible. Minor irritants like drumming fingers on the table, belching, tuneless whistling, rudeness, and cursing will eventually stop if you ignore them. Avoid giving them a big reaction. Sometimes the best response is no response. Of course it's hard to ignore behavior if:

1. It's harmful to your child.
2. It's destructive.
3. It really gets on your nerves.

When parents resort to punishment, they often fall back on scolding, yelling, and spanking. They wait until their child's behavior is intolerable, and then they lose their temper. In a sense this works, at least briefly. The child quiets down, and the parent is reinforced for losing control. Unfortunately, when parents lose control and punish a child in anger, the child doesn't remember what he was punished for. What he does remember is the pain and humiliation of being yelled at.

There are punishments that work. But unfortunately most parents don't make good use of them. Instead they are provoked into using the wrong punishment at the wrong time.

---

[13]Patterson, G. R., & Reid, J. B. (1970). Reciprocity and coercion: Two facets of social systems. In C. Neuringer & J. Michael (Eds.), *Behavior modification in clinical psychology.* New York: Appelton-Century-Crofts.

Marge Wilson is in the kitchen cooking supper for her two girls. In the next room, the noise level has been building steadily for the past twenty minutes. Three-year-old Robin runs into the kitchen complaining, "Amy stole my Barbie!" Amy shouts in from the other room, "Your Barbie is behind the couch, stupid!" Mrs. Wilson says to the younger girl, "Momma's busy, Robin, please go in the other room and stay away from Amy if you two can't play nicely. Amy, leave your sister alone, please."

Two minutes later, there is a loud crash in the next room and Robin starts wailing. Mrs. Wilson runs into the room as Amy is saying, "I didn't do it! She fell off the chair!" Mrs. Wilson shoves Amy aside and goes over to her younger daughter. Robin is more shaken up than hurt, but now both daughters are crying and Mrs. Wilson is shouting at them to "Please be quiet!"

This mother waited too long. Instead of dealing with a problem before it got out of hand, she waited until she lost control. She could have interrupted the escalating teasing by sending one of the girls upstairs or bringing one of them into the kitchen to help her. She could have used a mild punishment as soon as it became clear that Amy was teasing her sister and that the two girls weren't going to settle things on their own.

If you decide to use punishment, stay calm. Although punishment seems antithetical to responsive listening—because the emphasis is on being punitive rather than being understanding—effective punishment is applied without argument, without nagging, and without lecturing. The message isn't "You did something bad and you are a terrible kid" but rather "Sorry, but this is the consequence for that behavior." Use something mildly unpleasant, but do it before you lose your temper. Be consistent. Also reinforce desirable alternatives. For example, each time Mrs. Wilson sees her daughters playing peacefully together, she could go over and say, "Hey, that's really nice. You two were playing so quietly I hardly knew you were there. What are you doing?"

One of the most effective forms of

Behavior patterns don't change overnight. Be patient—but be consistent.

punishment is *time out*, which works as well with school-age children as it does with younger ones. "Time out" means time out from reinforcement. Reinforcement refers both to activities the child would like to be engaging in and to social stimulation, which of course includes arguing. You can put a child in time out by having him sit in a chair for five minutes with nothing to do, or by sending him to the bathroom or to his own room.

> "I told you not to keep banging on the table, but you disobeyed me. So I think you need a time out. Come over here and sit in that chair until I tell you that you can leave. I'll let you know when your time is up."

Five minutes works about right. Some people advocate telling children how long their time out will be, but not doing so keeps the control with the parent and eliminates a possible subject for argument.

> "Mom, it's been five minutes. Can I come out now?"

> "No, it's only been four minutes and fifty-eight seconds. You can come out when I tell you."

> "Mo-om, you said five minutes!"

Putting a child in time out should eliminate arguing—which is why scolding and lecturing are generally ineffective forms of discipline. At the end of five minutes (or so) just say, "Your time out is up now." Don't say, "You can come out and play."

If a child refuses to go to time out, the parent should escort the child physically. Even if the child is kicking and screaming, the parent should usher the child into his room or the bathroom, put the child inside, and close the door. If necessary, the parent should stand by the door and hold the handle until the five minutes is up. If the parent is firm, eventually the child will learn that there is no use fighting the time out.

Whether you decide to use time out or some other form of punishment, remember that positive reinforcement works better than punishment and that reinforcing a positive alternative often works better than punishing a child for doing something you don't like. If you apply punishment, do so deliberately and calmly and as soon as possible. (This is one reason why grounding is second only to nagging as an ineffective form of punishment with school-age children.)

Deciding to use punishment doesn't mean there's no room for communication and no need for understanding. Be sure to explain to your children why you're punishing them and be open to hearing their side of the issue. Responsive listening doesn't necessarily mean negotiating or failing to follow through with your efforts to enforce limits. Being sympathetic doesn't make it harder to enforce the rules; it makes it easier.

There is a reason for every misbehavior. Understanding why your child does what he or she does is half the battle of knowing how to control it, or in some cases knowing that you can't control it. Take your child aside, take a deep breath, and listen to his or her side of the story. You want to hear what was happening at the time the incident occurred, what led up to it, what happened afterward, and how your child feels about what happened.

A word of warning. You'll probably have to convince your child that you're really interested in understanding why he did something you don't like and how he feels about it. When they misbehave, children expect to be rebuked. Be careful with "why" questions. Children expect "why" questions to be rhetorical (because they usually are). "Why are you doing that?" usually means "Stop it." One way to get past your child's assumption that you aren't really interested is to tell her that you really are. Another little trick is just to avoid the "why." "You want to go to the mall because—?"

Teaching by Example

"*Do as I say. . . .*" Most parents concentrate on explaining things as a way to teach their children. But the truth is, children learn more from modeling, from observing and copying what they see, than from listening to lectures. The expression "Do as I say, not as I do" is a testament to its own futility.

A few years ago, basketball star Charles Barkley touched off a controversy by saying "I am not a role model." What he meant was that children shouldn't look up to celebrities as models to emulate. But people don't choose to be role models. Children imitate the behavior of adults they see as powerful and whose actions are rewarded. Few adults occupy a more powerful position in a child's life than his or her parents.

Furthermore, at least as far as children are concerned, parents do pretty much whatever they want around the house.

Unfortunately, one of the things parents model is being argumentative.

Whenever either of her children says something to her, Mrs. Neidemeyer asks for details.

> "Mom, Tommy got kicked off the soccer team, and now I'm the starting sweeper!"
>
> "Why did Tommie get kicked off the team?"

Unfortunately, Mrs. Neidemeyer's questions often reflect her own interests and not necessarily her children's. Instead of listening receptively to what her children are trying to say, her questions wrest the conversation away from what the child was trying to communicate. She's not really arguing, but she's not really listening, either.

Do You Contribute More Than You Realize to Arguments with Your Children?

None of us likes to think of ourselves as argumentative, but the truth is that most of us have a few habits that contribute more than we realize to family arguments. Take the following highly unscientific quiz to start thinking about things you might be doing that feel like arguing to your kids.

How Argumentative Are You as a Parent?

Do the following descriptions apply to you:

1—Rarely?   2—Sometimes?   3—Often?

_____ 1. When arguing with your child, you are careful to avoid bringing up problems that happened in the past.

_____ 2. When your child is being stubborn, you use criticism to break through the stubbornness.

_____ 3. When your child shifts from the issue at hand to criticizing

you, you are careful to confine your own comments to the issue at hand.

_____ 4. When your child describes something that you didn't witness,
you try to understand what the child is communicating rather
than interrogate him or her in a way that might make the child
feel doubted or challenged.

_____ 5. You recognize when your child starts to feel under attack, and
at that point you stop arguing.

_____ 6. When your child argues, you make a point of hearing him out
before challenging or refuting his position.

_____ 7. You explicitly acknowledge your child's point of view in an
argument before countering with your own.

_____ 8. You acknowledge the legitimacy of your child's wishes even
when you don't agree to what he or she wants.

_____ 9. When your child tells you something, you show your interest
by asking questions before trying to acknowledge what the
child is trying to say.

_____10. If your child thinks you said one thing but you think you said
another, you admit that you may have forgotten rather than assuming that you know what was actually said.

_____11. Family members have complained that you have a tendency to
go on and on about things.

_____12. When you criticize your child, you keep going until he or she
acknowledges what you've said.

_____13. When arguing with your child you make a sincere effort to
understand what he or she is saying rather than just waiting to
respond.

_____14. After an argument with your child, you are more likely to try
again to explain your position than to acknowledge your
child's position.

_____15. You feel free to express your critical opinion of your child's
choice in clothes.

Scoring: Add the scores you assigned to items 2, 9, 11–12, and 14–15; then
reverse the scores you assigned to items 1, 3–8, 10, and 13 and add this
number to the first score.

A score of 31 or over suggests that you tend to be very argumentative.

A score between 21 and 30 suggests that you are about as argumentative as the average parent.

A score of 20 or less suggests that you are less argumentative than the average parent.

Parents of argumentative children often fail to see that much of their children's behavior is a mirror image of their own actions. They're more aware of their children's response than they are aware of how they come across. Arguing is the product of an adversarial atmosphere. Parents contribute to an adversarial atmosphere by automatically questioning instead of listening to what their children say and by disputing whatever their children say.

It may be difficult to avoid speaking harshly when your children are disobeying. But an angry tone adds to the adversarial atmosphere. The more you respect your children's feelings, the more they will respect your authority. Talk with, not at, your children. Be conscious of your attitude and tone of voice:

Tell the truth.
Keep complaints specific.
Be careful with criticism.
Stop yelling.
Don't nag, don't lecture, and avoid advice.

Some parents say that their children listen to them only when they raise their voices. That may be true, of them. Perhaps they don't mean business until they yell. Then the yelling is a signal to the child that now they mean business, but it nevertheless serves to create an adversarial atmosphere. Better to speak softly and yet still be firm. Your words—and your follow-through—can signal that you mean business, and this way you avoid generating anxiety, and the contentiousness that goes with it.

When children complain that their parents are too busy arguing or lecturing or asking questions to hear their side of things, they're telling us why they feel the need to argue. When your parents don't listen to what you try to tell them, arguing may feel like the only way to get heard.

CHAPTER 8

Teenagers

"YOU CAN'T TELL ME WHAT TO DO!"

For teenagers, life is simple. All you have to do is stand by while your body, raging with hormones, shoots up, changes shape, and sprouts hair in the most unlikely places. Well, not exactly stand by. Just finish high school and figure out what to do with the rest of your life; fall in love and have your heart broken at least once; shed old friends; make new ones; and transform yourself from the child you were to the adult you want to be. Oh, by the way, sex is death and rain kills fish.

Freud called the years from when children enter school to adolescence *latency*, not because they are uneventful but because they have a steady sameness. Kids at this age do more for themselves and spend as much time as possible with their friends. Meanwhile, their parents, facing middle age, are rediscovering their own lives: reevaluating their careers, and maybe their marriages; trying to find time for friends; worrying about money; and dreaming of a vacation. Preteens need their parents less, and parents have more time to themselves. It's the calm before the storm.

The storm is called "adolescence": a time of unequaled turbulence, when anguished parents watch their good-natured little children turn into smart-mouthed, sullen teenagers. Arguments now take on a new dimension. No matter how contentious young children are, parents can usually count on having the final say. This is not true with teenagers.

Most parents can learn to listen responsively to younger children because they know they can enforce their wills once the conversation is over. Young children accept that their parents are in charge. They know that what they are allowed to do depends on what their parents decide. That's why young children are grateful to be listened to. They appreciate the opportunity to say what they want even though they may be disappointed by their parents' ultimate decision not to let them do what they want.

What makes responsive listening harder with teenagers is that they are no longer grateful for your willingness to hear their opinions. They now *expect* to be listened to.

When Karen got tired of arguing with her son Jonathan about what time he had to come home, she said, "No, you can't stay out past 9 o'clock on a school night, and that's final." As far as Karen was concerned that was the end of the discussion.

But Jonathan wasn't ready to give up. "That's so stupid! Why do you have to ruin everything I want to do!"

Jonathan was arguing not only to stay out later but also to be treated with what he thought of as a sense of fairness. As far as he was concerned his mother was being arbitrary.

But to Karen, Jonathan's criticism felt like a lack of respect, and so, understandably, she got mad. "I won't have you speaking to me that way, young man! You're grounded for a week."

Jonathan stomped out of the kitchen and went into his room and slammed the door. There he brooded over how unfair his mother was, how she never let him do anything, how she never listened to his side of things.

Two days later, Jonathan's friend Will invited him to stop by after school to see his new dirt bike. Jonathan, who knew his mother would say that he should come straight home, told her that he had to stay after school for band practice.

At 6:30, when Jonathan got home, his mother was waiting for him in the living room. An hour earlier Jonathan's friend Isaiah, who plays trumpet in the band, stopped by to ask if Jonathan could come over to study. When Karen asked Isaiah why he wasn't at band practice, he said there wasn't any band practice. So much for the honor system.

Karen was furious at Jonathan's lying to her. She told him that he was now grounded for two weeks and that he wouldn't be allowed to watch TV or use the telephone.

When he first walked into the house and saw the look on his mother's face, Jonathan felt guilty for lying to her. Now he just felt angry at her for overreacting. Alone in his room with nothing to do, he felt like a prisoner, and he thought of his mother as his jailor. *Why was she so mean? What's the big deal about going over to a friend's house? I don't do half the things other kids my age do. I don't smoke pot. I don't even smoke cigarettes. Okay, so I lied to her, but the only reason I did was because she's so unreasonable.*

Meanwhile Karen decided that she could no longer believe what Jonathan said. If he was going to lie to her, she was going to have to stop trusting him. She was going to have to keep tabs on where he went, who he talked to, for how long, et cetera. Unfortunately, the more Karen cracked down, the more Jonathan started sneaking around. Forced into a role she never wanted, that of her son's jailor, Karen also began to feel like a prisoner.

Control-and-Rebel Cycles

Most teenagers go through a period of rebelliousness, defining themselves as independent through opposition to their parents. Signs of defiance begin early.

Byron Meeks recalled that when his daughter, Allisa, turned twelve she began taking a tone that he found hard to accept from his little girl. The first time he noticed this change was when Allisa was looking for her red barrette and asked him if he'd seen it in the family room.

He couldn't find it and said, "No, honey, I don't think it's in here."

"Then where the hell is it!" she snapped.

Byron was speechless. It wasn't the "hell," it was that tone.

These early signs of disrespect are one of the harbingers of adolescence, and the parents' response is critical. Most parents understand that a certain amount of defiance is normal in adolescents, but while they learn to tolerate some insubordination, every parent has his or her limits.

A mother may be willing to put up with her daughter's sarcasm but not with her wearing too much makeup to school. A father may be willing to ignore his son's calling one of his teachers an asshole, but not when his son turns that kind of language on him.

When their teenagers exceed the limits of their tolerance, parents get provoked. They react emotionally, and their first impulse is to crack down.

> "What's that on your face? You look like a tramp! Get yourself upstairs, young lady, and wipe that gook off your face. I won't have you going to school looking like that."

> "What did you call me! Don't you ever use that word with me again as long as you live!"

Such reactions, meant to be educational, are about as instructive as a slap in the face.

Most parents underestimate the influence of their own actions on their children. Parents of adolescents worry about how to cope with rudeness and disrespect, but they have a hard time recognizing that much of what their children do is in response to what they do. What they miss is the *reciprocity* of the relationship.

Parents see their dear sweet little ones turning into ornery adolescents. What they overlook is their own failure to accept their children's growing autonomy. What's really ornery is the adolescent's insistence on growing up.

Preadolescents begin to argue about everything and anything—short skirts, baggy pants, tattoos, R-rated movies, junk food, taking out the garbage, messy rooms, homework, grades—you name it. Predictable battles take place over whatever parents are most anxious and insistent about. A mother with few friends may nag her daughter to invite other kids over to do something together; a father who didn't get much education may pester his son into defiance over homework. A boy whose father is a health nut may define his independence by smoking like a chimney.

The real issue isn't really friends or homework or health habits; the problem is that teenagers are challenging the rules that govern their relationship with their parents. When they look in the mirror, they may not be sure exactly who they are or who they want to be, but they know who they *don't* want to be: They don't want to be their parents. And they no longer want to be their parents' little darlings, either. Therefore they resist both imitation and obedience. Unfortunately, most parents tend to overlook the circularity of these struggles: More control triggers more rebellion.

Like their parents, teenagers prefer to think of themselves as autonomous individuals. But as with any relationship, that between parents and children is more than an association of separate persons. A relationship is an organic thing with a life and rules of its own. It is a mutually constructed system, in which the two halves that make up the whole begin to define each other.

One of the most powerful dynamics in any relationship is *accommodation,* the process of mutual adjustment by which two parties shape each other into a complementary unit. Accommodation is the reason intimate partners lose some of their individuality in becoming A Couple—a single, hyphenated unit of him-and-her. When you walk beside someone for a while you tend to coordinate your steps.

Accommodation helps to explain why stepparenting can be so difficult. A mother and child, or father and child, get to be like long-married partners in the sense that they gradually adjust to each other's temperaments and tolerances. The child will learn, for example, when the parent is serious and when he or she hasn't quite gotten to that point. The parent will learn that obedience doesn't always have to be automatic or instantaneous. But a new parent, who hasn't been part of this process of accommodation, may expect to impose his or her expectations on a parent-and-child system whose members have already accommodated to each other.

Arthur was a widower who remarried when his daughter Cathy was twelve. Arthur's new wife, Adrienne, took to the role of stepmother with energy and enthusiasm. She took Cathy shopping, helped with her homework, and took more of an interest in her comings and goings than Arthur had ever had time for. But with this involvement came a tendency for her to criticize what she saw as Arthur's permissiveness and Cathy's lack of discipline.

Arthur thought Adrienne was a little too bossy and, moreover, that her tendency to bail Cathy out when she got into trouble only contributed to Cathy's failure to take more responsibility for herself. However, when he tried to say anything to Adrienne, it always ended up in a huge fight. He'd say something like "I think we should back off a little," at which Adrienne would get furious and launch into a tirade. As a consequence, Arthur spoke less and less to Adrienne about Cathy and retreated more and more to the sidelines. Adrienne felt that, after turning over the responsibility of Cathy to her, now all Arthur did was criticize her. His silence didn't fool her.

When Arthur called me for a consultation, I suggested that he bring Adrienne and Cathy. I was surprised when he showed up alone. "She's *your* daughter," Adrienne had said. "You go."

After Arthur explained the situation to me, I pointed out that in any triangle there are usually two people who are close and a third who is distant. The best way to reduce conflict, I said, was for him to move toward both his wife and his daughter, separately. The closer he got to each of them, the less preoccupied they would be with each other. I explained how he could use responsive listening to minimize his tendency to get into arguments with each of them. I asked him to try this for two weeks and then bring his wife and daughter to our next meeting.

Once again, Adrienne refused to accompany her husband to our session, but Arthur had gone to the trouble of keeping a diary of his attempts to use responsive listening.

He had begun by initiating a conversation with Adrienne in which he made a concerted effort to empathize with her position. "Honey, I've been thinking about our tendency to argue about Cathy, and I think I need to try a little harder to understand your point of view. You think we should be a little stricter with her, don't you?"

"I suppose you think we should ignore her rudeness, her lousy grades, and the fact that she does *absolutely nothing* to help out around here! You always take her side against me."

Arthur hated the way Adrienne turned everything into an accusation. But he remembered what I'd said about responsive listening, and he was determined to try to sympathize with his wife's feelings. "I'm sorry," he said. "I guess you've taken the brunt of Cathy's defiance, haven't you?"

"Well, it's true, isn't it?" she said.

When you make the effort to use active listening with someone who's angry at you, you might expect them to be grateful. "Oh, thanks for being so understanding." But often the first sign that your listening is working is the expression of more anger. Don't react. Catharsis is a sign that active listening is working.

"You feel like you're the only one making an effort with Cathy, and that all I do is criticize you for it?" Arthur offered.

"Well, who cleans up her messes? Who makes sure she does her homework? And who takes her to school when she's late? I don't see you doing any of those things."

"I know I should be more involved. And I know that I haven't always let you know how much I appreciate how much you've done with Cathy."

At this, Adrienne softened. Instead of her usual attacking, she began to talk about how unhappy she was, how worried about Cathy, and how alone she felt. Once Adrienne shifted from attacking Cathy to talking about how overwhelmed she felt, Arthur found it easy to sympathize with her.

Talking to Cathy turned out to be a little easier, and a little harder. The easy part was sympathizing with her feeling that Adrienne was overly critical. The hard part was not taking sides. When Cathy complained, "She's *always* picking on me!" Arthur felt inclined to agree with her. But he knew that would be a mistake.

"It hasn't been easy for you, has it, honey?"

"How come *she* gets to decide everything about what I should do, and how come you always take *her* side?" Cathy was angry at her stepmother's intrusiveness, but what hurt most was her sense that the father she loved had abandoned her.

It's never easy for a parent to listen to a teenager's accusations of unfairness. Once this would have been Arthur's cue to defend himself, but now he just listened. "I'm sorry, honey, I know we haven't been as close as we used to be."

"Why do I always have to listen to *her?*" Cathy said. "You used to be so nice, but now I just get bossed around all the time. You don't even care," she said, on the verge of tears.

Now Arthur didn't have to pretend to be sympathetic. "You wish it could be like it used to be, don't you?"

"No," Cathy said. "But I wish I could talk to you more."

Previously, Arthur had felt that he had only two choices, either to challenge his wife's criticism and his daughter's defiance or just to stay out of it. Now he was finding that responsive listening gave him a tool to move closer to these two women he loved without getting into an argument. It wasn't easy for him to remember that you can understand someone's feelings without having to agree or disagree with their opinion. What Arthur learned was that making a stepfamily work is like succeeding at any other activity. You have to put in the hours.

When accommodation breaks down, the other great dynamic in relationships takes over—*polarization*—in which even slight differences magnify each other.

As with accommodation, polarization can be conscious but often occurs outside of awareness. A mother might decide to be a little more lenient with her children to compensate for what she sees as her husband's excessive strictness. Or a teenager might make a point of buying her clothes in thrift shops in order to be as different as possible from her Ralph Lauren mother. In both of these examples, the polarization may be intentional. But while some of the controlling and rebelling that goes on between parents and adolescents is deliberate, some of it just sort of happens.

When her son Scott decided that he was too old for hugging, Arlene turned more of her attention to her younger child, Kimberly. Scott was jealous of Kimberly's easy affectionate ways, but watching his little sister cuddle with Mommy made him embarrassed about his own dependency needs. And so without either of them thinking much about it, Scott's declaration of independence pushed his mother into a more affectionate relationship with Kimberly, which stiffened Scott's resolve to behave with what he thought of as a manly disdain for tenderness.

The same impulse that moved Scott to reject his mother's embrace also drove him to reject whatever opinions she might express. The ensuing arguments were predictable. If Arlene said that a particular rap song was crude, Scott defended its poetry and passion. If Arlene said that soccer looked like fun, Scott said it was a stupid game for wimps who couldn't play football. These disagreements were annoying enough, but when it came to more personal issues, like Arlene's opinion of Scott's friends or feelings about how he was spending his time, the arguments turned nasty. The more Arlene expressed reservation or disapproval of anything that Scott considered his prerogative, the more determined he became to defy her.

Arlene was tired of all the arguments. But she was afraid to relax her grip, afraid that Scott was too immature to exercise good judgment in the wide world of adolescent temptation. The more Arlene tried to hold him back, the more Scott hurled himself into the mosh pit of adolescent experimentation.

Polarization can be a subtle matter of two people nudging each other in opposite directions, or, when it comes to parents trying to control a teenager's independence, polarization can be as subtle as a train wreck.

Parents who worry about their adolescents making bad judgments miss the point that children don't learn to make judgments without practice. How many parents want their children to grow up depending on others, no matter how wise, to make their decisions for them?

The point of teenage rebellion isn't to reject what your parents tell you to do; it is to reject *that* they tell you what to do. Adolescent rebellion isn't a rejection of parents; it's a rejection of dependence on them. Parents who respond to these autonomous strivings by increasing their control only increase their children's need to resist.

Control-and-rebel cycles are a form of polarization in which two sides react to each other by increasing the intensity of their own response. It's an automatic and, in a sense, mindless process, the product of reactive emotion. Teenagers don't want their parents to control them with restrictions; parents don't want their teenagers to control them with defiance. As a result, both sides are driven to greater extremes—in almost knee-jerk reaction to each other's actions.

More control provokes more rebellion—and more rebellion provokes more control.

Once a pattern of polarization is entrenched, it can be activated by either the parent or the child.

Parents who think of their teenagers as defiant confuse autonomous strivings with stubbornness. Most teenagers are strong-willed, not oppositional. They struggle not to defy their parents but to achieve a measure of self-determination—and they struggle with as much effort as it takes. How far they carry that struggle, how extreme their behavior, is determined largely by how tenaciously their parents insist on trying to maintain control.

A girl who can't win control of how she dresses for school may express her independence by putting on Gothic makeup after she leaves the house. If she can't win that battle, she may escalate further, deliberately coming home late or getting into shouting matches with her mother. Or she may choose to defy her parents by smoking cigarettes or shoplifting or experimenting with drugs. Reckless experiments, chancy relationships—all for the honor of being her own person. The irony is, of course, that the defiant teenager isn't being her own person; she's being exactly what her parents don't want her to be.

The most common ways to break this commandment are setting inflexible standards; insisting on having the last word; and dictating to teenagers without giving them a chance to express their opinions.

The first commandment for parents of adolescents should be Thou shalt not become a force against which to rebel.

Silent Arguing

Ellen Berman walked into the living room where her son Freddy was sprawled on the couch watching a rerun of "Friends." "Honey," she said, "tomorrow is recycling day. Will you please put out the recycling bins before you go to school in the morning?"

"Uh huh," Freddy said.

The following afternoon when Ellen came home from work, she was annoyed to see that Freddy hadn't put out the recycling. She was angry, not only because she hated to see the garage filling up with bottles and newspapers, but also because Freddy had broken yet another agreement with her.

As should be obvious, Ellen didn't really have an agreement with her son. She asked him to do something, and he mumbled whatever it would take to get her to leave him alone. Freddy might not have intended *not* to take out the recycling. But, on the other hand, he never really made a conscious commitment to do so.

Although some teenagers rarely argue with their parents, they don't exactly do what's asked of them, either. They agree only to avoid being hassled. Their "Okay" doesn't so much mean "Okay, I'll do it" as it does "Okay, I hear you, now leave me alone."

Boys may use this strategy more than girls. Teenage boys tend to avoid ver- **Silent arguing is the** bal confrontations for the very good rea- **teenager's secret weapon.** son that they can't handle them. They get too upset. Research suggests that men and boys have greater diffi- culty tolerating arguments because they become more physiologically aroused than women.[1]

You can recognize silent arguing in a persistent pattern of not liv- ing up to what you thought were your child's responsibilities and by a general avoidance of discussion. When confronted, the silent arguer will say "I forgot" or "I was going to do it later."

Maybe the teenager who never cleans his room doesn't think it's fair to have to. After all, it's his room, isn't it? Even if you don't agree with your child's reasons for ignoring your requests, he may feel a whole lot more like complying if you acknowledge those reasons.

When a child (or anyone else for that matter) repeatedly fails to do what you expect, it's a safe bet that he doesn't want to do it. That much may be obvious. But what may be less obvious is that silent arguers of- ten "don't get around to" something because they don't think that par- ticular something really needed to be done—or don't think that they should have to be the one to do it. One way to find out is to ask.

"It seems like I'm always having to get after you to clean your room. Do you resent the fact that I make you straighten up your bed and put away your clothes?"

"*Mom*—I told you I would do it. Just let me finish watching this program."

Asking a teenager why he doesn't do what you ask isn't as easy as it sounds. When a parent asks, "Why haven't you cleaned your room like you promised?" or "Why don't you ever take the garbage out when I ask you to?" a teenager is likely to assume that these are rhetorical ques- tions. Let's face it, they usually are.

If you really want to find out why a silent arguer doesn't do what

---

[1]Gottman, J. (1999). *The marriage clinic: A scientifically based marital therapy.* New York: Norton.

you expect, you have to convince him that you're really interested in how he feels. A good way to invite these feelings is to ask your child if the reason he doesn't do a particular chore is because he doesn't think it's fair. Then be patient and wait for the answer. It may take time to convince your child that you really are willing to listen.

The main reason for arguing silently is not believing that the other person is open to your point of view.

"No, I didn't mean that you should do it now. I'm really interested in whether or not you think it's fair for me to decide how you should keep your room."

"Well, if you really want to know, I don't see why I should have to make my bed. It's my room, isn't it?"

Once you get a silent arguer to start expressing his reasons for not complying, you have two options. You can let him know that although you understand how he feels, he still has to do what you ask. Or you can compromise. That's up to you. But whatever you decide, why not take some time to think it over?

"Well, maybe you have a point there. Let me think about that, and I'll talk to you again tomorrow."

In any kind of business negotiation, responsive listening is a power-ful device for overcoming opposition. If you want to sell somebody something or get him to do things your way, the best strategy is to first get him to express all the reasons he doesn't want to. Once you've heard and acknowledged his point of view, it no longer operates as an unspoken barrier to hearing what you have to say. The most effective strategy to winning someone over is to start by hearing his side.

You can use this same strategy to get your kids to stop using passive aggression to avoid doing what you ask. But do you really want to deal with your children as though strategizing to outwit an adversary? Or do you want to use responsive listening to help your child learn to express her feelings and argue for her point of view? If you stop to think about it, do you want your children to go through life being unable to argue for what they want and not knowing how to stand up for what they be-lieve in?

Remember: It isn't an agreement just because the other person says "uh huh." It's only an agreement when the other person really agrees to do what you're asking. How do you tell the difference? You ask.

Suppose you didn't just settle for a mumbled "okay." You actually got your teenager to explicitly agree to do a certain chore, but then he still doesn't do it. Then what? If this question resonates with you, give some thought to the likelihood that you're still having trouble with the idea that people don't do what they say they'll do for a reason. Until these reasons are expressed, heard, and acknowledged, they will continue to operate as forces of resistance.

But there is an even more important reason that teenagers often don't do what their parents expect of them. Because they no longer accept the idea of obeying authority without question, the most effective way to reach workable agreements with adolescents is through *negotiation*.

Negotiated Agreements

Responsive listening with younger children is intended primarily to allow them to express their feelings. Parents of school-age children still have firm control over the decision making, because children at this age accept that their parents are in charge. With adolescents, responsive listening shifts to allow teenagers more input into decisions.

Negotiating, rather than dictating, allows parents to resolve issues—about curfews, house rules, clothing, hairstyles, dating, and so on—with less conflict. It also fosters a greater willingness on the part of teenagers to cooperate with the rules. A negotiated agreement is a real agreement.

When adolescent children aren't involved in the decision-making process, they're rarely committed to the final decision. Since their feelings remain unexpressed, they end up silently criticizing and passively resisting.

The subtext in much of the arguing that goes on between parents and teenagers is: Who is going to define the rules of the relationship? Teenagers are no longer willing to accept a relationship in which the parent controls the decision making and expects the adolescent to obey "because I said so." Instead of having power struggles over who controls whom, it's better to redirect this energy by involving the adolescent in the decision-making process.

> **The surest way for parents to squander their authority is to make rules that teenagers don't agree to and that can't be enforced.**

The principles of negotiation are simple. Both sides state their positions, and then they work out a compromise. Unfortunately, this process often degenerates into arguing. The surest way to turn a negotiation into an argument is not to acknowledge the other person's position. Saying something like "Yes, but . . ." is how this usually works.

"You can go to Nancy's party, but I want you home by eleven-thirty."

"But the party isn't over until one!"

"Yes, but I don't want you out past midnight."

"I finished mowing the lawn. Can I go over to Brian's house?"

"Yes, but you didn't trim the hedges."

"Come on! Why don't I get to have any fun on the weekend?"

"That's not true! You have lots of free time. I don't think that trimming the hedges is too much to ask."

Responsive listening is the antidote to the three greatest sources of resentment that adolescents have toward their parents:

Their parents don't listen to them.
Their parents don't respect them.
Their parents aren't fair.

What makes these complaints more understandable is realizing that adolescents expect to begin to control their own actions, while their parents may still expect to dictate to them as children.

Parents can demonstrate respect for their teenagers' feelings by explicitly emphasizing the issues of fairness and respect.

"You can go to Nancy's party, but I want you home by eleven-thirty."

"But the party isn't over until one!"

"Do you feel it isn't fair for you to have be home before the other kids?"

"It *isn't* fair."

"If I let you stay out a little later than eleven-thirty, what would you suggest?"

"How about one?"

"Now *you're* not being fair. I'm trying to compromise, and you aren't showing any willingness to meet me halfway."

"All right. How about midnight?"

Teenagers respect fairness, especially when it's reciprocal.

"I finished mowing the lawn. Can I go over to Brian's house?"

"Yes, but you didn't trim the hedges."

"Come on! Why don't I get to have any fun on the weekend?"

(*Deep breath*) "Do you sometimes feel that I don't respect how hard you work at school all week?"

(*Shocked silence*) "No. I feel like you think all I do is sit around and talk to my friends."

Note: This is the beginning of a real conversation. When you use responsive listening to invite your teenager to complain, don't expect him or her to thank you right away. The real sign that the channel of communication is open is when your teenager trusts you enough to complain about a perceived lack of respect or fairness.

With responsive listening, a parent shows respect for an adolescent's opinion by asking for it—and taking it seriously. In studying what adolescent girls value most in their relationships with their mothers, Harvard professor Carol Gilligan found that daughters appreciate their mothers listening to their ideas, mothers sharing their own feelings, and relationships changing as a result of give and take, with daughters being more willing to listen to their mothers' suggestions after having had a chance to express their own ideas and opinions.[2]

While some daughters describe their mothers as authoritarian, daughters also describe themselves as unyielding: "We don't like to admit that the other is right. I go, She might be right and I may believe what she is saying, but I won't say it."[3]

It is this readiness to resist control that responsive listening is designed to overcome. Children are more likely to cooperate with agreements that they've had a hand in negotiating. They get to say what they think is right, their parents have their say, and the final agreement is a compromise worked out between them. But what sounds simple in principle is often anything but simple in practice.

If parents prove unwilling to compromise, teenagers soon see "negotiations" for what they are: a sham, just another parents' trick for imposing their will.

"I won't let you go to the movies on Sunday afternoon if you haven't finished your homework for Monday."

This isn't a contract. There was no negotiation.

"If you want to go to the movies, what do you propose doing about your homework?"

"I'll do it after I come home."

"By the time you get home from the movies it'll be time for supper."

"Okay. How about if I finish all my homework before we go to the movies. Then can I go?"

"Sure, that's fine."

Why go to all the trouble to come up with such a simple and obvious solution? Because the child came up with it. If the parent had imposed it, the teenager would feel resentful and be less motivated to live up to it.

But even if parents are willing to negotiate in good faith, these discussions often break down in the face of emotionality. When emotions heat up, it isn't possible to negotiate productively. When a negotiation

---

[2]Gilligan, C., Lyons, N. & Hanmer, T. (1990). *Making connections: The relational worlds of adolescent girls at Emma Willard School.* Cambridge, MA: Harvard University Press.

[3]Gilligan and colleagues (1990, p. 265).

deteriorates into an argument, parents should drop the idea of trying to reason with their children and just listen. If that becomes impossible, break off the conversation and resume it later.

When discussions become heated, the person who knows how to use responsive listening is way ahead of the game. But knowing when to switch from negotiating to just listening—and remaining cool

> **What fuels arguments are counterarguments; what defuses them is hearing what the other person has to say.**

enough to do so—can be extremely difficult. A better strategy is to be proactive instead of reactive. Instead of waiting for disagreements to crop up, parents can circumvent a lot of arguments by initiating discussions about family rules before they become issues.

Set aside time to be with your children and encourage them to bring up wishes and complaints. This kind of initiation produces a whole different atmosphere.

The same proactive spirit can be applied to brainstorming discussions of family problems. For these sessions to have any value, parents must convince their children that the discussion isn't just a pretense for making them do what their parents wanted them to do in the first place. In brainstorming sessions, when someone comes up with an idea, no one should criticize it. Keep track of all suggestions. Usually someone criticizes each idea. The net effect is that people stop coming up with ideas, and they feel devalued. Some of the "suggestions" made will be

> **dialogue (n.): the free flow of ideas and opinions between two or more people. Parents who are skilled at dialogue make it safe for their children to add to the shared flow of ideas, even if their ideas are at odds with their parents' ideas.**

little more than emotional catharsis—but by not arguing with them, the negotiation doesn't deteriorate into a quarrel.

A Certain Amount of Control

Now the bad news. You can't eliminate arguments with adolescents just by listening to their point of view. You win only by being willing to lose a little. Or to put it another way, only by giving up on the idea of complete control can parents retain a certain amount of control over their teenagers. And, with teenagers, *a certain amount of control* is all that's reasonable to hope for.

If you've told your son a thousand times not to leave dirty dishes around the house, but he keeps doing it anyway, maybe you should let it go. Maybe it's better to give up on some things—even if "It's not right!"—than to continue to play the role of constant critic, a voice against which your children learn to deaden themselves.

The only way to retain parental authority is to gradually let go of trying to control everything about your adolescent's life.

In practice, relaxing control means negotiating instead of dictating, giving up on some things, and giving in a little on others. To quote the president who came between Lyndon Johnson and Gerald Ford, "Let me make one thing perfectly clear": I can't tell you what rules and regulations you should let go of. Oh, I could tell you, but you'd be a fool to listen. Every parent has to decide such things for him- or herself—or, if there are two parents, for themselves.[4] What I can tell you is that if you don't learn to let go of some things, you will drive your child into more rebellion, overt or otherwise.

Most teenage disobedience involves deception.

But having acknowledged that I can't tell you what rules to enforce, I can make a suggestion. Don't fight with your kids about *how* they speak to you. Trying to control a teenager's language leads to a lot of unnecessary battles. I don't know about you, but I don't recall cursing around the house when I was a teenager. I'm not sure it was a matter of anything my parents did to control it; we just didn't do that when I was a kid. Today's teenagers have grown up with less authoritarian control than previous generations. As a result they are mouthier and less deferent, especially at home.

Accept your teenager's right to say what he or she feels, no matter how rude or unreasonable it seems.

---

[4]The questions are endless, and none of the answers are easy. They depend on personal values and preferences, and the right answer varies with the circumstances. Do you let your teenage daughter drive your new car? How responsible has she shown herself to be? Does she do her chores and keep up with her schoolwork?

Bear with me a minute while I tell you a story that may not seem to have much to do with teenagers. A prosperous horse breeder once consulted me about problems in his marriage. This was one of those May–December matches between a wealthy older man and a beautiful young woman. At first it was an idyllic relationship, but then, after a few years, they were on the verge of divorce.

"I just don't understand what happened," the man said with obvious pain. "We used to get along so well. Then, somehow, she just changed. . . ."

When he met her, she was a waitress, recently divorced, working to support her two-year-old daughter.

"She used to be so sweet. We were always together. She shared my love of horses, and she was so helpful around the stables. I don't understand what happened. She changed."

It's easy to see this man's mistake. He couldn't adjust to his young wife's gradually wanting to have more independence, to spend some time with her own friends, and not always to be at his beck and call. But don't parents often make the same mistake with regard to their children?

> "Ginger used to be so sweet. She used to give me cute little cards with smiley faces on them. She was so helpful around the house. She always asked if there was anything she could do. I don't understand what happened. She changed."

Yes, she changed. It's called growing up. But with teenagers, it's not *being* grown up; it's struggling *to* grow up. Teenagers are in transition from childhood to adulthood. In the process, they must redefine not only who they are but also who they are in relationship to their parents.

You do not win the battle for control with teenagers. Those things that parents absolutely don't want their kids doing—drinking, smoking marijuana and taking psilocybin, having sex, cutting school, hanging around with bad company—most teenagers are going to experiment with no matter what their parents say or do. Actually, it's a little more complicated than that.

The adolescent's parents are already a part of him or her, in the form of a developing conscience. It is this inner voice that now begins to exert the most powerful influence on an adolescent's decisions—but not if parents are controlling or punitive. We think about what's right or wrong only when we don't have somebody standing over us, telling us what to do.

"Yes, but," one parent asked, "how do you balance the need to know what's going on in a teenager's life so that you gain information that may protect the child with the need to allow the child autonomy and privacy? What's acceptable and not acceptable to have hidden from you as parents? How do you communicate that to the teenager?"

Very good questions, but I'm trying to be descriptive, not prescriptive. What I'm trying to describe is that parents who don't begin to relax their attempts to control their teenagers only tend to provoke more rebellion. And I'm suggesting that teenagers generally keep secret those things that they suspect their parents might give them a hard time about. Draw your own conclusions.

How do you gain information necessary to protect your kids from dangerous activities outside the house? You can make a habit of asking them where they're going, who they're going with, what they're going to do, and what time they'll be back. But these questions are useful primarily to let your children know that you're interested and that you care. You can't control what your teenage children do.

Suppose you have some outside information about something your child has done that he's either kept secret or lied about. Do you talk to the child or keep the information to yourself?

I can see going either way with this. By not telling your child what you know, you avoid embarrassing him or her. But secrets from people you love are a heavy burden. Not telling is, of course, your secret, and it is a form of lying.

Sometimes when you're not sure whether to bring up an awkward issue, you can tell the other person your dilemma. In this case that might go something like "There's something I'm not sure whether or not I should talk to you about. It's something that I found out about you, but I'm afraid that if I bring it up you'll feel like I'm checking up on you. On the other hand, I don't want to pretend that I don't know."

When you tell someone that you're unsure whether to discuss

something with him, curiosity will usually prompt him to tell you to go ahead. But by describing what you're afraid might happen in the conversation tends to make the other person avoid responding in the defensive way you feared he might.

Although some parents squander their authority by trying to control what their teenagers do out of sight, most of the usual arguments take place over things parents can see, like taking out the garbage and putting their dirty clothes in the hamper or what time to come home at night. Parents can cut down on arguments without giving up their influence by recognizing that although they may not be able to control their adolescents' actions, they can influence their decisions.

Teenagers may not want to be controlled like children anymore, but their parents' approval still matters to them. Disapproval, not control and not punishment, is the most powerful form of influence parents can wield over their adolescent children. When teenagers break the rules, their parents should confront them with what they did and say that they don't like it. This is often preferable to threats, lectures, and punishments. It's hard to argue with "I don't like what you did."

When teenagers break the rules, parents can cut down on arguments by responding with:

1. A clear statement that the rule has been broken.
2. Emphasizing that such behavior is unacceptable.
3. A declaration that the rule remains in effect.

"You stayed out way past your curfew last night. That isn't acceptable. I want you in at 10:30 and on time in the future."

"10:30 is way too early. It's not fair! None of the other kids have to be home then. You can't make me come home that early."

"That's right, I can't make you. But that's when I want you home."

"I don't care."

But they do care. And the 10:30 curfew will continue to exert pressure on her every time she goes out.

Children risk nothing by *saying* that they will disobey their parents' orders. They may not actually be willing to defy their parents, but they lose nothing by saying that they will.

Just Drop It

"Sandy, have you seen my gold earrings?"

"Uh, they might be in my room."

"I thought I told you that I didn't want you borrowing my good jewelry."

"I forgot."

"I don't want you taking my things without my permission!"

"Mo-om! I didn't have anything to wear to Randi's party, and you weren't here."

"Why can't wear your own earrings? I gave you a perfectly nice pair for your birthday."

"Why are you always nagging me? Why can't you just leave me alone!"

"Don't you talk to me that way, young lady."

"You can't tell me how to talk."

"Don't you dare talk back to me!"

Et cetera. Et cetera.

Why not:

"Sandy, have you seen my gold earrings?"

"Uh, they might be in my room."

"Thanks."

Or if that's too hard:

"Sandy, have you seen my gold earrings?"

"Uh, they might be in my room."

"Thank you, Sandy. But please don't take my good jewelry again. I've asked you not to before."

"I forgot."

Finis.

Arguments don't end until somebody has the last word—or is willing to let somebody else have the last word. Parents may have good reasons for insisting on getting their message across, but if your aim is to communicate something about the issue at hand, the best thing to do is to say your piece and then shut up. By going on and on, parents convey only one thing: that they insist on being in control. What they say counts. What their kids say doesn't count. And so the issue shifts from the matter at hand to a battle of wills.

The easiest way to control who has the last word is to let the other person have it.

Wait a minute! "Let the other person have the last word"? Surely that's easier said than done. Yes, it is.[5]

Putting adolescent rebellion into context means seeing it as part of a polarized pattern, propelled by the adolescent's rejection of authoritarian control, and by parents' failure to adjust to the teenager's growing need for autonomy. But this analysis focuses mainly on behavior and, as we shall see, polarization has as much to do with perceptions as with actions.

In the Mind's Eye

Life is complicated, so we find ways to explain it. These explanations, the stories we tell ourselves, help us to make sense out of our experience and justify our behavior.

"Of course I yelled at him. He has no respect for anything I say."

When parents come to see their teenagers as "rebellious" or "defiant," they not only leave themselves out of the equation but also begin to develop tunnel vision, which leads them to notice and remember only those events that fit the Rebellious Teenager story line.

Thus, a mother who comes to see her daughter as "demanding and inconsiderate" will remember all the times her daughter stayed out late or

---

[5]For a set of easy-to-follow steps for avoiding trying to get in the last word in arguments with people who push your buttons, send a million dollars in cash to me care of the publisher of this book.

needed a ride at the last minute, and she'll tend to forget the times when her daughter helped cook supper or volunteered to wash the dishes. Each of the daughter's demands confirms the mother's story line that, like other important people in her life, her daughter doesn't really care about her feelings. The daughter, in turn, is acutely aware of how often her mother refuses to give her a ride to the mall or criticizes her for wanting to spend time with her friends. Thus, she gradually develops a narrative around never being able to satisfy her mother, which makes her give up caring about what her mother thinks. Both mother and daughter remain stuck in a cycle, not simply of control and rebellion but, more specifically, of noticing only incidents of control or rebellion.

Such closed and rigid narratives make parents and children reactive to each other and quick to argue, as the following example illustrates.

Ruth's daughter Abby wants to sleep over at her friend Linda's house on Friday night.

"I don't want you sleeping over at someone's house on Friday. I want you here." Ruth defended her decision with indignation, as though her daughter's request were part of a pattern of selfish disregard for anyone but herself.

Abby's face reddened. She had been ready for a fight, and sure enough, here it was. "Why not?" she demanded. But it didn't matter what Ruth said in response. Whatever reasons her mother gave, Abby was prepared to shoot them down.

Ruth, who didn't really have any reasons and was now too mad at this latest incidence of her daughter's "inconsiderateness," could only sputter, "Because I don't want you to, that's why."

"Mom! What the hell—I can get a ride!"

"Leave me alone. I'm tired," Ruth said, her cheeks blotched with color. "Because we want you here Friday night. That's all."

"Why can't I see my friends!" Abby moaned. "I don't want to be here!"

Sound familiar?

Notice how this argument is driven by "totalizing views"—parent and child reducing each other to one set of frustrating responses. Abby isn't mad just because her mother won't let her sleep over at Linda's house.

She's mad because her mother Never Lets Her Do Anything. Her mother is Unreasonable, Bossy, Controlling, Unfair. Aren't all parents?

Likewise, Ruth isn't upset just because Abby wants to sleep over at her friend's house. She's angry because her daughter is Selfish. She's Inconsiderate, Demanding, Disrespectful. Aren't all teenagers?

Parents reduce their children to stereotypes when they see them only as objects in relation to themselves. The person who doesn't do what you want is, by definition, stubborn, right? Parents who see their teenagers as "stubborn" and "irresponsible," as though that were the sum total of their being, are likely to be seen in turn as "critical" and "controlling." When this happens, both sides start collecting grievances, saving them up like coupons. For what?

Is the not-uncommon parental view of teenagers as "lazy" a complete distortion? No, a lot of teenagers are lazy around the house. That's because home is the natural arena for expressing the dependent, childish part of themselves. The teenager's more independent and considerate side is usually on view only away from home, often unseen by his or her parents.[6]

The way to break the grip of totalizing views is to ask yourself, How does the other person prefer to think of herself? How does she prefer to be seen? Once you start thinking this way, you begin to see the other person's actions in a more reasonable light.

We've seen how the adolescent's rebelliousness is reciprocally related to the parent's controlling and how this control-and-rebel cycle is driven by the tendency of both generations to view each other in stereotyped, oppositional terms. Thus, we've gone from blaming arguments with teenagers on their rebelliousness to seeing these struggles as part of an interpersonal pattern, first in behavioral terms and then, adding a cognitive dimension, emphasizing that people's actions are based on their perceptions. But it's impossible to fully understand the polarization of parents and teenagers without seeing it in context with the need for the family system to evolve in order for children to graduate into adulthood.

> **When a teenager seems to be behaving "unreasonably," it may help to consider what would make that response understandable.**

---

[6]When your children get to be twenty or thirty-five, they'll still be teenagers when they come home to visit.

PART III

Complications

PART III

Complications

CHAPTER 9

The Changing Dynamics of the Adolescent Family

You don't have to tell parents of teenagers that their children are changing. Those slow to adjust their rules to accommodate their soon-to-be-adult children will find their hands full with arguments.

"What do you mean 'Be in by eleven'? That's ridiculous!"

"How old do you think I am?"

What may be less obvious is that adolescence is not only a transition for teenagers; it's a time of transformation for the entire family system.

The Myth of the Hero

We don't always think of families as systems. In fact, the coming-of-age drama is usually seen as a young person's struggle to break away from childhood dependence, to take hold of adulthood and the promise of the future. Much of the conflict between teenagers and their parents can be understood as a product of the search for identity and authentic selfhood. Above all, teenagers want to be masters of their own fate, heroes of their own stories.

We were raised on the myth of the hero: Superman, Wonder Woman, The Lone Ranger. When we got a little older we found real-life heroes: Martin Luther King, Eleanor Roosevelt, Nelson Mandela. These men and women stood for something. If only we could be a little more like these heroic figures, who seemed to rise above their circumstances. Only later do we begin to realize that some of the "circumstances" we wanted to rise were part of the human condition—our inescapable connection to our families.

The counterpart of the hero is, of course, the villain. Heroes need villains every bit as much as they need their shining armor. Teenagers are all too ready to see their parents as villains, stubbornly conspiring to stifle their freedom with rigid and antiquated rules.

Just as toddlers must give up the secure place on their parents' laps to explore the house, so must adolescents give up their secure place in the envelope of their families in order to venture out into the world of love and work. In the process, the adolescent becomes a critic—challenging parental beliefs, exposing hypocrisies, and undermining long-standing prejudices. Although it's possible for parents to accept this challenge as good for their children, and good for themselves, many parents feel threatened and fight back. This often begins an escalating series of conflicts, which in many cases are never settled, only broken off when the children leave home.

If parents are to remain heroes, albeit flawed heroes, of their own stories, they are hereby forgiven if they come to view their adolescent offspring as some combination of heroes and villains. Heroes or villains, the myth remains the same: In good times and bad, family life is seen as a product of intersecting personalities. One reason for blaming the turmoil of adolescence on those moody, ungrateful kids of ours is that it's hard to see past individual personalities to the structural patterns that make them a family—a system of interconnected lives governed by strict but unspoken rules.

The secure parent will grasp the fact of having become a target for the child's challenging self-assertion and will respond in a tolerant, respectful manner. When an angry teenager demands to know *why* he has to be home by midnight, an understanding parent will listen responsively to the child's point of view. When does *he* think he should be home? What is he planning to do? With whom? Then, after hearing the child's opinion, the parent will reconsider the rule—not necessarily change it, but not automatically stick to it, either—rethink it, taking into account the child's growing ability to make his own decisions, though reserving the final decision for the executives of the family. This is a shift from a complementary position ("Because I'm your father, that's why!") to a more symmetrical stance ("Because I worry about you; why, what's your proposal?"). What parents decide should make sense to adolescent children, even if they don't like it.

Sixteen-year-old Keith asks, "Dad, can I go skiing this weekend with Joshua?"

"Are his parents going?"

"No."

"Then you can't go. Sixteen is too young to go away for the weekend without adult supervision."

"Oh, come on, Dad, don't you trust me?"

"I trust you, but I also worry about you sometimes. And I don't like the idea of you boys driving all the way to the mountains on a snowy weekend."

"You say you trust me, but any time I want to do anything you always say no."

"Well, I'd be willing to let you go skiing, but not just you and Mike without someone older along. If his parents aren't going, do you have any other suggestions?"

"How about if Mike's brother goes with us, and he drives. Would that be all right?"

"How old is Mike's brother?"

"Twenty-five."

"Well, if he goes with you, I guess it would be all right. But I don't know Mike's brother and I'd like to meet him before I give you my final okay."

"I'll call Mike right now, and if his brother will go with us, can they come over now so that you can meet him?"

"That would be okay."

In this example, the father uses responsive listening not simply to acknowledge his son's feelings but to make room for him in the decision-making process. In being willing to compromise, this father let his son win, though he did so in a way that took his own concerns into account. Successful parents avoid power struggles with their children.

Sometimes listening to their feelings is enough, but sometimes *choosing* to compromise is the best and most reasonable way to retain their authority.

Earlier I said that adolescence is a time when every teenager has to discover his or her own personality. It is that, of course, but it's also a time for redefining the shape of the family.

Adolescence is a period of corrective derangement, in which every teenager has to remake his or her personality, and every family has to remake itself.

Healthy families have clear boundaries between parents and children. These families manage to balance closeness and independence, resulting in personal freedom as well as a sense of belonging. Unlike the rigid boundaries of disengaged families, a clear boundary is open enough to encourage communication between parents and children. But, unlike the blurred boundaries of enmeshed families, a clear boundary gives children room to grow and explore—and gives their parents room to pursue lives of their own.

When children reach adolescence, the boundary between generations becomes a little wider to allow teenagers the room for autonomy that they need to grow into adulthood.

Speaking of boundaries, wise parents cut down on arguments with adolescents by recognizing that the limits of their control end with the front door of the house.

Breaking Away

Adolescence is about letting go and taking hold. Letting go of dependence on parents and taking hold of life outside the family are reciprocal achievements. Success in one sphere facilitates success in the other. When parents are locked in struggles with their adolescent children and look for ways to "solve" these problems, they might do better to back off and do what they can do to support their children's involvements outside the family.

Arguing with your parents may not be a lot of fun, but sometimes it beats the anxiety of being independent of them, of being on your own.

In real life nothing much happens, although everything is considered. In fantasy, where adolescents spend considerable time, everything is possible. Teenagers are tormented by restless sexuality, on the one hand, and, on the other hand, their own guilt about having "dirty thoughts." One minute they're transfixed by the latest video by Britney Spears—all wet-lipped and tarty. The next minute they're ashamed of themselves for being such slaves to sexuality.

Sexuality isn't, of course, the only thing teenagers struggle with. They must also work out who they are, what they want to look like, how much to give in to guilty pleasures like smoking and drinking and drugs, and whether to join their friends in flaunting authority by shoplifting, getting tattooed, or dropping out of the competition for college. One reason asceticism holds such appeal to the adolescent imagination is its power to blot out guilt and shame. Teenagers want to make the world a better place, and they want to purge themselves of unholy appetites. They're seeking reasons and meaning in life, and they're building the structure of their own personalities, controlling the unruly upsurge of sexual and aggressive impulses.

They dream of becoming missionaries and take refuge in books with idealistic heroes like Anne Frank or Holden Caulfield. Some stop eating meat ("the flesh of animals"); some stop eating almost everything.

Most teenagers are anxious and uncertain about their bodies, though in our culture girls still suffer the most over their appearance. Parents may try to argue—"You look fine!"—but reasoning is at best irrelevant, at worst counterproductive. The problem is that teenagers are all too ready to battle with their parents rather than face their own internal conflicts.

Here's a little secret about human nature: the most troublesome conflicts are often projected. The five-year-old who fights with his mother (or father) often turns out to have a father (or mother) who's angry at his wife (or husband) but afraid to fight openly with her (or him). The real conflicts may be about intimacy or independence, but it's easier to argue over how to raise the children. Likewise, the man whose wife "won't let him have any fun" probably has his own issues about "self-indulgence." The thirty-year-old who can't seem to stop battling authority figures is likely to have unfinished business with a domineering parent. Whenever you see conflict that seems to be neurotically stubborn, it's worth considering that it might be displaced.

Teenagers argue with their parents to get their way, of course, but also to avoid having to resolve their own conflicts over obedience and guilt, pleasure and virtue, self-indulgence and self-denial. Children cling to battles with their parents as a way to avoid letting go of their childish selves. They manage this by becoming experts at baiting their parents into prolonged and repetitive arguments.

It isn't the family that the adolescent struggles to disengage from but his or her childish ties to it. These struggles are played out within the adolescent and between the adolescent and his or her parents. The struggle takes place primarily with the parents when the adolescent externalizes what he or she is unable to tolerate internally as conflict, anxiety, guilt, shame, or depression.

Adolescents, who struggle with an upsurge of hormonal drives, aggressive as well as sexual, seek a target of their unruly impulses in the environment. Different adolescents express these primitive emotions in various ways, but one of the most common forms of projection is the adolescent tendency to fight with their parents as a defense against falling back on their own childish dependency.

Parents are, of course, not immune from being provoked into arguing back in the face of their teenagers' verbal assaults. See if you can provide a typical parental response that the following adolescent provocations pull for:

"I don't care."   _____

"No, I won't!"   _____

"I will if I want to."   _____

"You're an asshole!"   _____

(This is one of my favorites. First, because people in my generation can't imagine having said that to our parents. Second, it's a way to get parents going even when you can't think of a thing to say about the issue at hand.)

If you came up with . . .

"We'll see about that!" or "Well, then, maybe you won't care if I ground you for a week."

"Yes, you will" or "I'm warning you."

"No, you won't" or "You do, and you'll see what happens."

"What did you say?" or "Don't you dare talk to me that way!"

Congratulations, you could be a card-carrying parent.

How do you avoid getting hooked into becoming a stand-in for a teenager's displaced conflict? The same way a fish avoids getting hooked by an angler. By not rising to the bait.

Why Don't They Say What They Mean?

Not rising to the bait is, of course, easier said than done. Teenagers are masters of the put-down. It's a skill they develop sparring with their friends, where they learn to protect themselves against painful feelings of being uncool by cutting other people down to size. With other teenagers, they can be direct with their mocking comments. In case you haven't noticed, kids can be very cruel to each other.[1] But when teenagers use mockery with their parents, they don't always say exactly what they mean.

What they say:	*Translation:*
"Whatever—"	"That's stupid, and I wish you'd stop nagging."
"Chill out."	"Don't get so upset; you're acting like a fool."
"Okay, Mom."	Politer version of "whatever," meaning, basically, "Leave me alone."
"Yeah, sure, Dad."	"That's ridiculous, and you're an idiot."
Sarcastic look.	"You are beneath contempt. But I don't dare talk to you directly about what I think."

---

[1]Maybe the people who make Prozac should develop a drug to obliterate all memories of the seventh grade.

These comments and the sneering looks that go with them can be very hurtful. But it's hard to defend yourself against these zingers because they are rarely direct enough to cross the double line. Why don't teenagers say what they mean? Because they're afraid of how their parents would respond if they were more direct. Hard things usually get said indirectly.

What do you do when your teenager gets snotty with you? You can counterattack, you can walk away, or you can talk about it. Counterattacking is, unfortunately, the most common impulse, and it's part of the symmetrical pattern that fuels arguments. If I were a strategic therapist, which I'm not, and I wanted to suggest a sneaky reversal, which I would never do, I might suggest that instead of fighting back when your teenager puts you down you start crying.

I favor strategy number two. When somebody hurts my feelings, I walk away. I get very quiet, and I stay that way for two or three days. This strategy, technically known as pouting, must be a good one because I learned it back in the good old days, when I was about four.

Alternatively, when your teenager puts you down, you can talk about it—though not necessarily at the moment it happens. I don't know about you, but right after somebody says something hurtful to me I'm not very good at talking calmly about what happened.

Talking about what happened shows your child that you don't have to take potshots at each other; you can talk about what's bothering you, you can communicate. The most direct thing you say when somebody hurts you is "That hurts."

Suppose, for example, that you're trying to show that you appreciate your daughter's taste in music and she mocks you for it. "Oh, right, Mom, like you're so cool." You feel rebuffed and hurt. A direct and honest response might be "You know it hurts when you treat me like that. I have feelings, too, you know."

Similarly, when your teenager tries to catch you out in contradictions, inconsistencies, not practicing what you preach, or any number of other dreadful flaws (often as an excuse not to do anything you ask), it hurts, and most of us feel like striking back. You can resist the urge to do that by getting in the habit of reporting your feelings. "It makes me feel bad when you pick on me like that." Make sure that you don't pass off a counterattack as an expression of your feelings. "I feel like you're a stupid jerk for saying things like that."

What I've suggested is avoiding rising to an adolescent's bait and turning a dig into a fight by telling him when he hurts your feelings. But remember, you're the parent. You can do more than avoid fighting back. You can use responsive listening to find out what's behind your teenager's sarcastic comments.

"Do you feel like I've been unfair?"

"What do I do that makes you feel like getting back at me like that?"

Again, remember that you'll have to convince your child that you really are willing to listen to and consider the answer to such questions if you hope to find out what's going on.

Letting go and taking hold also describe the parents' challenge when their children reach adolescence. Parents must accept that there are now things in their teenagers' lives that they as parents no longer have control over. Most of the drinking, smoking, sex, and drug taking that adolescents do takes place outside the home, out of sight. Parents who try too hard to control these things end up in a lot of unnecessary arguments, or drive their children into lying and sneaking around.

The "letting go" that I'm advocating refers to the illusion of control, not to caring. Parents who fail to ask their children where they're going, who they're going with, and what they plan to do there may communicate that anything goes or that they don't care.

Letting go for parents of adolescents doesn't mean that you stop caring or that you don't keep open the lines of communication. It does, however, mean losing the little children who have been at the center of your life for a dozen years or so, the children you could cuddle, who told you everything, who wanted nothing as much as spending time with Mommy and Daddy.

Letting go means letting teenagers suffer the consequences of their own actions. If they don't get themselves up in the morning, let them deal with being late for school.

Adolescent rebellion serves a dual purpose: By arguing with their parents, teenagers are demanding respect for themselves as independent people, and they are readjusting family boundaries.

If we look at the family as a system in transformation, we will see teenagers in the vanguard for change. In pushing for autonomy, they are attempting to loosen their ties to the family and to redefine the rules of their relationship to their parents.

Parents are reasonable. They understand the need for change, *slow* change. Teenagers are impatient. One minute they're reasonable, the next minute they're high-strung and hysterical. Their push for autonomy polarizes their parents into pulling harder to maintain family cohesion and to enforce the old rules. Conflict is almost inevitable because parents want to slow the transition ("If only they'd be more responsible") and teenagers want to speed it up ("If only they'd trust me more").

For teenagers to correct the narrow reality of the family, discover dormant potentials in themselves, and win the esteem of their friends and respect of their teachers, they must venture far enough to be exposed to wider realities. Children must be secure enough in their parents' love that they neither try to please them by always doing whatever they want nor defy them by always doing exactly the opposite.

Young children idolize their parents and draw strength from closeness to them. Adolescents repudiate their parents—or at least blind allegiance to them—and pull away in order to find strength in themselves. Self-respect demands that they prove to themselves that they are capable and don't need their parents to direct their lives. "*Please,* Mother, I can do it myself!"

The sudden reversal of adolescent feelings toward their parents is a measure of how urgent the need is to create distance where once there was a need for closeness. This withdrawal—repudiation, really—is still felt as a loss by teenagers. It causes them considerable sadness and pain.

The child's contradictory needs for distance and closeness are reflected in an unpredictable alternation of emotional withdrawal and emotional hunger. The same teenagers who reject their parents as hopelessly out of step still need them. One minute they're stubbornly set on doing things their own way, the next minute they're all uncertainty and doubt. "Mom, what should I wear?" Empathy, following their moods, is easy at this stage, like following a drunk driver on an icy road.

Staying Connected

Eileen Carlson, age forty-one, is married with six children, ages three to seventeen. Although all of the children keep her busy, most of her arguments are with Darren, fifteen, her second oldest. He picks on the younger children and his mother. If his brother Robby (eleven) or sister Chelsea (eight) has trouble or is slow to do something, he'll call them dumb or stupid. Naturally, this name calling makes them cry, and then his mother has to intervene to protect them, saying something like "Darren, be quiet!"

"Darren picks on everybody," his mother says, "even adults. He thinks of it as clowning around, but he often carries it too far."

One of the things that annoys Eileen most is Darren's habit of pestering her when she's busy trying to cook supper. He'll stand too close and bump her while she's trying to work. If she tries to ignore him, he'll persist, trying to outlast her. Now she's less patient and will tell him to leave her alone. When she gets mad, she'll yell at him or spank him with a wooden spoon. But now that he's older and bigger, Eileen usually turns to her husband to discipline Darren.

Even though Darren is now fifteen, it seems that he still wants his mother's attention. For all their opposition to parental authority and breathless enthusiasm for the adventures of the youth culture, adolescents still need their families. Family is a refuge to return to from time to time when they get discouraged, hurt, or simply worn out.

Darren's arguments with his mother are a good example of the self-perpetuating nature of many family problems. Eileen's answer to Darren's pestering is to ignore him, and then, when she finally loses her temper, to punish him. When this doesn't work, she does what most of us do with solutions that don't work: She tries more of the same.

What Eileen might try is responsive listening. When Darren crowds around her while she's cooking supper, she might ask some specific questions about what he was doing that day.

"How did soccer practice go today?"

"What is that new math teacher like?"

"Did you do anything interesting at school today?"

Darren's wish to still be close to his mother—on his time and terms, naturally—is echoed by a surprising number of teenagers.

Sixteen-year-old Trevor lives with his mother, stepfather, sister, and half brother. He's going into the eleventh grade.

"In my family, we all go to church together. That's the only time we're together. My mom cooks Sunday dinner, but we all eat at different times. I'm usually outside until after everybody else eats, and then I eat in front of the TV.

"My mom and I used to be close, but now we don't say too much. My mom will come and say, 'Hi, how was your day?' But not very often. I wish she did it more.

"I don't think my mom knows what's going on in my life. I don't show her who I am. I try to talk sometimes, but sometimes she doesn't want to hear me. My mom and I don't fight much. I guess that's because I stay out of her way. The only time we argue is when I want to go somewhere on the weekend, and she doesn't let me. She doesn't think I do enough—like homework and stuff around the house. I want to have a little fun. I don't think she knows how hard high school is.

"I know my mom loves me, but she doesn't give me enough attention. She used to, when I was younger. She doesn't notice if I'm upset or happy. My mom doesn't give me a chance to get a word out. Every time I try to, she interrupts and starts talking at me. Can't she just ask me, how was my day, what did I do in school? I want to talk to her. I don't ever talk to anybody in my family."

Trevor misses the closeness he once had with his mother, but he doesn't blame her. In fact, he is acutely aware of how hard it is for her to get up early and go to work every morning. Most teenagers are more aware than you might think of the financial and emotional pressures on their parents. This sensitivity can make it harder for them to turn to their parents for support, emotional or otherwise. When teenagers talk about their feelings about their parents, you hear a mixture of frustration and longing.

Whitney is fifteen. She lives with her mother and younger brother. "Ever since my father left, there was never any family time set aside. By the time I was ten, I started making my own plans, going with friends here and there and all around. My mom was always rushing around working and dating, dragging us to church or to her boyfriend's house.

We always had dinner sitting down together. I liked it, I guess. We talked about stuff at the table, but nothing important. When I was twelve or so, we would argue and argue because I'd want to do stuff with my friends and my mother would never let me. Dinner time became argue time. Now, whatever love I get, I get from my friends."

In order to hear what their children are saying, parents need to recognize that teenagers need space *and* closeness. Sound confusing? It's less so if you keep both of these needs in mind and take your cue from your children. The twin tasks of adolescent development, achieving identity and intimacy, are, in fact, coordinate achievements. Independence is requisite to real intimacy, and the answer to the question "Who am I?" depends in part on knowing that you can love and be loved.

How does a child whose parents give him or her both space and support experience adolescence? It's still a time of turmoil and confusion, but the child anchored in an accepting family faces this turmoil with a sounding board, a testing place, a home base. Having a stable supportive family makes it easier to venture out into the world, knowing that home is a safe harbor to return to when necessary. At the same time the adolescent is forging an individual identity, he or she also retains a sense of belonging—a family identity.

To some parents the idea that their adolescent children still need them may ring false. Their complaint is "My teenager never talks to me."

The Vanishing Act

When teenagers start avoiding their parents and not having much to say when they are around, parents feel rejected. It hurts to be shut out.

"Just once I'd like to be able to sit down and have a conversation with him. I don't think I'm being unreasonable."

Teenagers avoid talking to their parents to protect themselves from prying and criticism. This reticence can be understood psychologically, as part of the adolescent's need for privacy, and interpersonally, as a product of the teenager's relationship with his or her parents.

As long as parents think of their teenagers primarily as objects in relation to themselves—rude or polite, cooperative or uncooperative—instead of as independent persons in their own right, it's easy to forget how much pressure they live with.

Teenagers, those noisy, strutting adolescents who prowl the shopping malls, wearing baggy pants and lip gloss and thumbing their noses at convention, live under terrific stress. Imagine growing up in a world where a terrorist attack might occur at any time, sunbathing causes cancer, making love can lead to the fatal AIDS virus, your parish priest might turn out to be a child molester, pollution is burning a hole in the earth's atmosphere, and acid rain is poisoning all the lakes and streams. These aren't easy things to contemplate when you are fourteen or fifteen.

Today's teenagers also live with incredible pressure to succeed, and it starts early. Competition for admission to the best schools begins with preschool, and it doesn't let up. By the time they reach high school, most middle-class children are subject to enormous pressures to get As, do well on the protean SATs, and cultivate extracurricular activities—whether they want to or not—in order to get into the right colleges. And, of course, today's teenagers have to cope with what teenagers have always had to cope with: the torment of self-consciousness.

Exposed and trapped in their own bodies, under scrutiny all day at school, preoccupied and troubled by sex, adolescents feel conspicuous and vulnerable. In response to this heightened feeling of exposure, they turn inward. When you ask them what they're thinking, they say, "Nothing." They retreat from visibility. They long for privacy.

Teenagers retreat to the privacy of their rooms to soothe themselves and deal with their hurts. In the morning they wake up, exiled from their dreams, into the raw world. In the evening they want to relax, to escape from anxious pressures. They seek release from vexation and vulnerability by getting away from the eyes of others, getting lost in their music, and entering the world of dreams. What they *don't* want to do is talk about what they did in school today.

> **We all need privacy at times. The reason adolescents need it so badly is that revolutionary changes in their physical and psychic selves make them feel terribly exposed.**

"But they talk to their friends," you might say. Well, yes, but their friends listen.

When parents complain that their kids never talk to them, it usually turns out that the children make overtures but the parents admonish, preach, teach, reassure, argue, challenge, and ask too many questions. In response, the kids slowly start pulling down the curtain that separates their inner life from their parents. Communication, or lack thereof, is always a two-way street.

It saddened Sheila that the closeness she'd had with her daughter up until the eighth grade had given way to a wariness on Becky's part about speaking openly. Sheila was doing her best, however, to keep open the lines of communication and to avoid letting their relationship degenerate into the endless string of quarrels that seemed to define her relationship with her sixteen-year-old son, Elliot.

When Sheila gets angry with her thirteen-year-old daughter, she keeps the argument from escalating by walking away. While she's cooling off, she writes down what happened in order to gain some perspective. Later, maybe after supper, she'll go back to talk it over. Here, for example, is how she described one recent run-in.

When Becky continued to receive CDs she hadn't ordered from a record club, Sheila reminded her that she needed to write them a letter. Becky's brother Elliot, who happened to overhear, wanted to know "A letter about what?"

"It's a 'Mom letter,' " Becky replied disdainfully. The implication was clear. The letter wasn't Becky's obligation, it was another of those annoying things her mother unreasonably insisted on.

"That's a lie," Sheila said, none too calmly. "It isn't my problem; it's hers."

"Oh, Mom," Becky said, "I was just joking!"

"You're *so* funny," Sheila said and went into the kitchen.

Later that evening, Sheila, who was a little embarrassed that she'd gotten so upset, went to talk with Becky about what had happened. "I felt really unhappy about that conversation," she said. "That business about it being a 'Mom letter' was completely untrue."

"Mom, I told you, it was just a joke!" said Becky.

"Watch your tone," Sheila warned.

Becky shut up and listened as Sheila explained, very calmly, why it was Becky's obligation to write the record club a letter and how she'd felt when Becky mocked that obligation. Becky nodded, but about all she said was, "Yes, Mom."

I hope that by now it's obvious what was missing from Sheila's attempt to reach an understanding with her daughter. (It's always easy to figure out what other people are doing wrong.) For all her well-intentioned efforts to avoid letting arguments escalate, Sheila's attempt to communicate with Becky after they both calmed down wasn't really very effective. Her mistake was trying harder to explain her own position, rather than trying harder to listen to her daughter's.

Here's what Sheila might have said instead:

"I felt really unhappy about that conversation. I was upset, but, after I thought about it, I realized that I didn't really understand your side of it, and I'd like to. How did you feel about what I said to you?"

Whenever you want to address a misunderstanding with someone, the following formula will help make it clear to the other person that you are now really willing to listen: (1) "I'm sorry about what happened; (2) I know how I felt, but (3) I realize that I didn't really hear your side of it, and (4) I'd like to understand your position."

It's possible that Becky's first response to this invitation might be just to try to drop the subject. An adolescent's reluctance to open up to her parents is based on her assumption that they probably aren't willing to listen to what she has to say. If so, Sheila could say something like "No, please, honey. I'm sorry about what happened, and I really would like to hear how you felt."

Listening responsively to teenagers means listening to what they're saying—even if it's "Leave me alone"—not making them say what you want to hear. Teenagers may not want to discuss certain things with their parents, or at least not until they're ready. Children avoid talking about subjects that are too personal or that make them feel vulnerable. There are moments, like at the end of a long day at school, when almost anything feels too personal to discuss. After five or six hours of being the object of close attention at school, teenagers often just want to be left alone. Their "nothing" isn't coy or withholding, it's self-protective. They're telling you that the subject makes them feel more vulnerable than they want to feel. Respect the child's boundary around the personal. Show interest, but don't press. If your child doesn't want to talk—show that you hear by backing off.

What children don't want to talk about has as much to do with timing as topic. Busy parents are eager to make the most of the precious time they have with their children. When they're together, they want to hear all about what's going on in the children's lives. But the kids may not feel like talking at that moment. You can't program "meaningful" conversation. Kids tend to talk seriously only when it's their idea. This usually occurs spontaneously, in the midst of everyday routine. That's why "quality time" is no substitute for being there.

You may be genuinely interested in what's going on in your children's lives. You may *want* to listen. But they don't know that. They expect that when their parents want to talk to them it's about checking up on them. If you want to break though a teenager's assumption that you're the warden, you'll have to convince him or her.

Ask questions that aren't likely to be taken as an interrogation. Ask questions that suggest your child's opinion is worth seeking out.

> "You took a course in ethics, Lucy. What do you think about letting the police search students' lockers for guns and drugs?"

Taken out of context that probably sounds like an honest question. But don't forget that teenagers are very sensitive to being asked questions that are nothing but a prelude for an adult imposing his or her point of view.

> "You took a course in ethics, Lucy. What do you think about letting the police search students' lockers for guns and drugs?"
> "I don't know, Mom."

The desultory answer doesn't necessarily mean "I don't want to talk"; it may mean "I'm not sure you're interested in listening." One way to ease someone into opening up is to start by asking one or two simple, concrete questions; they're easy and nonthreatening to answer.

"Have they instituted random locker searches at your school yet, Lucy?"

"No, they haven't. Why?"

"I read in the paper that they're starting to do that at a lot of high schools, and I was just wondering if they were doing that at your school and what you thought about it."

"I don't think they have any right to search our private lockers. Just because a few kids have been caught selling drugs doesn't mean that the rest of us should lose our rights."

You may have to prove to a reticent teenager that you're really interested in his or her ideas and opinions—which you can do so by choosing nonthreatening subjects, likely to be of interest to your child, and opening the conversation with a few simple questions. But when you show interest in the things they care about and a willingness to listen, almost anyone will open up to you.

Whether and when children feel free to open up to their parents depends on the reception they expect. If you demonstrate to your children that they can talk things over with you, without fear of judgment, they will. If you don't, they won't. If you accept your children's right to protect themselves with silence when they feel the need, and demonstrate understanding when they do express themselves, they will open up to you, in their own good time.

"Listening" to a teenager may suggest a goody-goody, I'm-OK–You're-OK dialogue, but it isn't always going to be that way. Sometimes what's on your child's mind will come out with a howl of frustration and rage. Sometimes he or she may have to scream, slam doors, and break furniture to even begin to describe what's eating him or her. Such raging and howling doesn't mean there is no dialogue. There is only no dialogue when you refuse to listen, when you don't try to understand.

Teenagers need practice to develop emotional literacy, the ability to articulate their feelings, to talk about friends, dreams,

If by some chance you want to turn a verbal outburst into an explosion, try the following: Don't listen, keep arguing, insist on getting the last word, and try to restrain a raging adolescent by blocking the exit when he or she has had enough.

wishes, frustrations, aspirations, worries, and anxieties over fitting in. Children who don't learn to put their feelings into words and don't have a responsive listener are handicapped in moderating their own internal emotional states. They don't know how to tolerate inevitable feelings of frustration, rejection, or anger. Without such internal resilience, kids turn to drugs, drinking, and sexual experimentation for soothing and distraction.

Adolescence is almost inevitably a difficult time for the whole family, but it needn't be as antagonistic and wounding as we've come to expect. It can be altogether more pleasurable, even exhilarating, for everyone in the family. The adolescent is a conduit to the world at large, bringing new styles, new attitudes, new information—even a new language—into the family. Adolescent children help keep their parents up to date; they keep their parents informed and they keep them on their toes. Often, however, the infusion of new ideas is unsettling.

The adolescent becomes a critic—challenging parental beliefs, exposing hypocrisies, and undermining long-standing prejudices. Although it's possible for parents to accept and appreciate this challenge as good for their children and good for themselves, many parents feel threatened and fight back. This often begins an escalating series of conflicts, which in many cases are never settled, only broken off when the children leave home.

Adolescence is the last chance for most people to put their relationships with their parents on an adult level. Those who fail to get beyond adolescent emotional reactivity with their parents will continue to react with similar knee-jerk emotionality to anyone who gets close enough to push the same buttons.

CHAPTER 10

When Arguing Seems Unavoidable

HOW TO USE RESPONSIVE LISTENING IN THE TOUGHEST SITUATIONS

If you give responsive listening an honest try, you'll find that it helps defuse potential arguments in a wide variety of situations. But you'll also find some instances in which it doesn't seem to work, or, although it might work, you find yourself losing your cool before you can put what you've learned into practice. Congratulations, you live in the real world, where there are no magic formulas. In this chapter, I'm going to describe a few of the circumstances that make it hard to listen and offer suggestions for how to deal with some of the curves children are so good at throwing their parents.

Instead of trying to organize this chapter in neat little themes, I'm going to begin with a few examples that raise questions about responsive listening. Let's see what themes emerge.

Six-year-old Olivia wants to sing to the grown-ups while they're having dinner. The other kids, having finished their pizzas, are watching a video. Olivia's dad, who's been trying to practice responsive listening, tells her to go ahead and sing. Olivia sings her song, and when she's done she wants to sing it again. Should her dad try responsive listening to find out what she really wants? Maybe she feels excluded by her parents or picked on by the other kids.

Should a parent who is entertaining friends use responsive listening to find out what's bothering his child? It depends. If Olivia seems especially unhappy, it might be nice to ask what she's feeling.

> "What's the matter, honey? Don't you feel like watching the movie?"

If a six-year-old is feeling left out and lonely, it doesn't hurt to take a minute or two to talk to her about those feelings. But it needn't take more than a minute or two. After that it's perfectly okay to tell her that now the grown-ups want to talk.

This is an example of how listening and limit setting often intersect. Healthy families have clear boundaries. Grown-ups have a right to time for themselves—and kids need to learn to stand on their own two feet. The basic principle of parenting here might be to teach a six-year-old that there are some adult activities that she will not be a part of. However, rule setting is usually more rather than less effective when it's preceded by a brief acknowledgment of a child's feelings. First asking the child what's the matter and then telling her to go and play is a responsive way to draw a generational boundary. Allowing a six-year-old to become the center of adult attention at a dinner party is blurring the boundary between children and adults.

Thirteen-year-old Christine and her father are constantly battling over her messy room. He asks her while she's watching TV to take a break during a commercial to go clean her room, and she gives him a withering look. He feels that what he's suggesting is reasonable, but she responds by being oppositional. How could responsive listening help Dad get what he wants and allow Christine to save face?

Okay, I have a couple of questions of my own, here. When does a child get to have the right to be in charge of how she keeps her own room? Thirteen? Sixteen? Thirty-five? Question number two: How do *you* like it when somebody interrupts you while you're engrossed in something?

The problem here is timing. If a parent wants to talk to a thirteen-year-old about her failure to do a chore, the best time to do so is when they're both calm and the child isn't busy doing something else.

To make responsive listening work, you may have to exert a bit of self-control. If you want to communicate, rather than just lay down the law, you may have to wait to address some issues until the right moment. In this example, the father might be advised to set clear rules and expectations. ("I want your room cleaned up tonight before you turn on the TV.") But, as mentioned earlier, when a child doesn't clean her room, it may be that she doesn't think she should have to. Use responsive listening to give her a chance to express her feelings on this matter. But choose a time when she may be open to talking.

Suppose your eight-year-old insists that you turn the radio off when you and your teenager want to listen to Eminem. Maybe the eight-year-old really hates the music, or maybe she just wants to control her environment, especially when she feels ganged up on by her mother and sister. How can you practice responsive listening with both children?

There are really two questions here. First, how do you decide what to do about the radio when the children disagree?

You realize that you, as the adult, are in charge, and then you decide any way you think best. Pick the choice you want or let the children take turns; it doesn't really matter, as long as you don't forget that you are in charge.

The second question—How do you practice responsive listening with both children?—is again a matter of timing. Some parents may be better able to listen to squabbling siblings in the car than I am—but I wouldn't even try. I'd give the kids a couple of minutes to work out their differences by themselves, and if, but only if, they couldn't, I'd settle it. I'd leave the responsive listening for how each of them feels about this until later when I could talk to them one at a time.

Here's a related issue: Can you practice responsive listening with one child and two parents at the same time?

It's important for parents to maintain a united front with their children. Sometimes this means making compromises so that the two of

you can be consistent; at other times it means speaking up to your partner about disagreements so that the two of you can work them out.
The most important thing is to be united and to support each other.
Sometimes two parents together can practice responsive listening effectively. But on issues that raise anxiety—yours, your partner's, or the
child's—it's easier for the child to talk to a parent one on one.

What about responsive listening when a child tries to play the parents off each other?

The real issue here is the parents' attitudes. When your child complains to you about the other parent, it's important to resist the urge to
use your child as an ally for your resentment against your partner (or
ex-partner).

Not only do children do best
with two parents who work as a
team, children also form their character by identifying with both parents—whether they want to or not.
Never undermine or criticize a

> **Some parents find it too
> painful to hate themselves for
> all their faults and failings;
> luckily, God sends a substitute,
> a husband (or wife).**

child's other parent to the child. And don't conspire against the other
parent by agreeing with the child's complaints about him or her. It isn't
necessary to agree with a child's complaints in order to be sympathetic
to his feelings.

How do you respond when your child complains about the other
parent? You play therapist. You listen and sympathize with the feelings,
but without saying that the child is right or that you agree—and certainly without adding complaints of your own.

How do you respond if you're a divorced parent and your child insists that your ex understands her better than you do? Same as above. (If
it hurts your feelings, seek solace from a friend.)

Mom comes home early and finds thirteen-year-old Denise and
two boys in the living room. They are listening to music on the computer. Nothing else seems to be going on. Mom is surprised, but not
completely. She says "Hi" and then asks the boys to introduce themselves. She doesn't blow up at her daughter, but Denise knows it's time
to send the boys home. After the boys leave, Mom says to Denise,

"This is not okay, and you know it. When you're home with boys alone, things can happen, even when you don't want them to. You need to find places to hang out with your friends that are okay, like going bowling or to the movies, or playing basketball, or something like that." Mom also asks Denise to explain how this happened.

Is this responsive listening or irresponsible parenting? Shouldn't the mom have laid down further consequences?

That depends—on whether she wants to teach her daughter to be responsible and obey the rules or vent her own anger. When a child is caught doing something she knows—and accepts—is wrong, she feels ashamed. In this instance, punishment, especially if it's harsh, typically makes children shift from feeling bad (about what *they* did) to feeling mad (about how mean *their parents* are). When it comes to punishing a child who probably feels ashamed of her actions, less is more.

There's an additional reason why in this example responsive listening is more important than punishment. Parents who want to set limits on their teenagers need to find out if their children think the rules they're asked to obey are fair. If they don't, the only way to control them is by becoming a full-time detective.

What comes out of these examples is a re-emergence of two themes we've touched on in earlier chapters. Responsive listening is intimately tied up with effective discipline and with respect for interpersonal boundaries in the family. But while firm discipline and clear generational boundaries make it easier to listen responsively, it can work the other way around as well—that is, the consistent use of responsive listening can improve these other areas of family functioning as well.

Discipline and Responsive Listening

Perhaps the example of Denise's mother who, when she found her thirteen-year-old alone in the house with two boys decided not to punish her, raised questions in your mind about discipline. Why shouldn't this mother have punished her daughter? After all, the child clearly broke an important rule, didn't she?

Effective discipline is partly a function of judgment and attitude. In her mother's judgment, Denise knew that she had done wrong by al-

Whenever possible, allow children to learn from the natural consequences of their behavior, which include feeling bad for doing something they weren't supposed to do.

lowing boys into the house, and she felt bad about it. Her mother correctly surmised that additional punishment might only make her daughter feel less guilty for what she had done and more angry at her mother for punishing her.

What I meant by saying that effective discipline is a function of attitude is that the parent who assumes she is in charge and acts that way doesn't hesitate to listen. She isn't threatened by what her children say. She's confident that she's the grown-up. She doesn't feel that she has to fight with her children over various issues: She knows what isn't worth fighting about, and she knows that she will win those battles that she decides are necessary to fight.

Imagine how you might approach spending a day as a substitute teacher for a class of eighth graders. Would you be worried? Hesitant? Insecure? Afraid that the children would get out of control and you wouldn't be able to do anything about it? Would you think it was your responsibility to make them sit still and be very good and polite? Would a Marine drill sergeant worry about this assignment? How would someone who liked and respected kids feel about this job? How would worrying about how the children would respond *to you* versus concentrating on what *they* might be interested in affect how the day went?

Feeling confident that you have the ability to control your children when you decide that it's necessary is far more important than worrying about this or that specific disciplinary technique. But feeling confident that you are in charge is only one element of your relationship with your child.

Listening and Interpersonal Boundaries

Many of the challenges to responsive listening that parents encounter relate to boundary issues. As you recall, clear boundaries between parents and children are sufficiently open to allow a free flow of communication but firm enough to keep children from certain adult activities— and to keep parents from intruding too much in their children's lives. Boundaries that are too rigid limit communication—and make parents less open to listening to their children's concerns. Boundaries that are too diffuse, on the other hand, make it harder to listen responsively because decision making is always open to debate and because it's hard to talk to an intrusive parent.

<blockquote>Children avoid talking about some things with intrusive parents because they don't want their parents telling them what to do—"giving advice," "making suggestions," and so on.</blockquote>

While it makes sense to say that the boundary between parents and children should be neither rigid nor diffuse, what constitutes a clear boundary is open to interpretation. Most of us take for granted the kind of boundaries we grew up with. What to do?

My advice is first to figure out if your own family was more enmeshed or disengaged. Enmeshed families are characterized by not closing bedroom doors at night, everybody getting in everybody else's business, parental concern about even the most trivial of children's activities, and very frequent visits and phone calls. There's a lot of communication, but not a lot of privacy or independent decision making. Instead of wrestling with hard decisions on the basis of what they think they should do, individuals in enmeshed families often make decisions based on avoiding disappointing other members of the family.

Disengaged families are characterized by more privacy but also by parents not knowing important things about their children, less open affection, infrequent visits and phone calls, and a tendency for individuals to keep things to themselves.

If you decide that yours was an enmeshed family, keep in mind that you may have a tendency to be intrusive, to expect to control more about your children's lives than necessary, and to have difficulty separating feelings from actions. If you came from a disengaged family, you may have a tendency to communicate less than you should.

The example of six-year-old Olivia, who wanted to sing to the grown-ups while they were eating dinner, is a boundary issue. Enmeshed parents might think they should allow a six-year-old to enter freely into this adult time. They would be open to her wish to sing—and slow to draw a line that says not to join in the grown-ups' dinner party. Disengaged parents would have no trouble keeping the child from intruding, but they might not take time to find out if she was upset about something.

Arguing with a thirteen-year-old who's watching TV about cleaning her room also raises a boundary issue. In my opinion, parents should allow children over about ten to decide how they want to keep their own rooms. But just as I wouldn't try to dictate to my children how they keep their rooms, I wouldn't try to dictate to other parents how they want to handle this issue. However, whatever chores you want your child to do, respect her enough to speak to her when she's not engaged in doing something else.

Some of the arguments parents have with children occur when the parents try to control what children see as their own prerogatives. Joanne, for example, doesn't want her daughter Alicia to study on the couch because "she's not comfortable on the couch."

Shouldn't that be up to the child? Parents who don't pick their battles blur the line between decisions that might better be left to the child and more important issues that the parents probably should decide.[1] Which are which? That's a judgment call. Just remember, if you come from an enmeshed background, think twice about what you need to dictate to your children. If you come from a disengaged family, you may have to get involved in issues—like whether school-age children do their homework—that may have been left up to you back in the good old days when you were a child.

One of the other examples we considered in this chapter involved the question of how to decide between two children's preference for what to listen to on the car radio. Although this wasn't the ideal example to introduce the subject (when will I learn to make up examples to suit my purposes?!), this scenario raises the question of how parents should deal with sibling rivalry.

Sibling Rivalry

Sibling rivalry is such a familiar term that it's become a cliché. The kids are fighting? Don't worry, it's only sibling rivalry. Tell that to parents whose lives have been made miserable by their children's constant arguing.

Why do brothers and sisters fight so much? Because they're jealous.

---

[1]Some parents attribute preferences to their children that they may not want to admit are in fact their own. If Joanne doesn't want her daughter to study on the couch for reasons of her own, saying so explicitly avoids blurring the image.

Older children are jealous of the young ones who come along to displace them; younger children are jealous of the power and privileges of their big brothes and sisters. So, a certain amount of resentment is natural.

Although parents wish their children wouldn't fight so much, it's a good idea to keep in mind that arguing is inevitable. Competition is natural, and it makes kids tougher and more resilient. Arguing teaches children how to assert themselves, defend their rights, and—if their arguments aren't interrupted—how, eventually, to compromise. Much depends, however, on the parents' response.

Many parents develop a repertoire of predictable responses to their children's quarreling, based on an intolerance of fighting and an exaggerated sense of the parents' duty to control their children. These responses, which begin by reasoning with the little adversaries and end with punishing them, interrupt squabbles before the children have a chance to settle them themselves.

The biggest mistake parents make in dealing with arguments between their children is not letting the children work out their own conflicts. Parents who try too hard to *teach* their children to get along cheat them out of the opportunity to *learn* to get along. Unfortunately, interfering parents get reinforced, at least temporarily, for interrupting arguments. Here's a typical example.

Just as the family is about to sit down for dinner, Adam and Matt start arguing about who is going to sit where. "I'm going to sit next to Daddy." "No, I'm sitting here." "No, me!" At this point, their mother interrupts. "If you're going to fight, go up to your rooms." The argument subsides, to be resumed later. They always are.

Avoid being an enmeshed parent by staying out of your children's arguments. Let them settle their own quarrels.

"Yes, but what if the children start hitting each other?"

Oh, they will. If they can count on you to intervene, they know that no matter what they do they will be safe. They can escalate with impunity. Once you start interfering, the kids will always run to you with their complaints—"Frankie hit me!"—and they'll never learn to negotiate as long as you insist on doing it for them.

To respect the boundary around the sibling subsystem, it helps to get clear about what belongs in their relationship with each other and what concerns their relationship with you. What time they go to bed, who goes to bed first, whether or not you will tolerate yelling in the car—these things necessarily involve you. Who calls who what in the backyard, who gets to sit in the front seat of the car this time, and the well-known Who Started It?—these things are their business. Let your children learn to negotiate with each other.

If your children start to argue or come to you with complaints about each other, the best thing you can do is to sympathize with their feelings, express faith in their ability to work it out, and leave the room.

"Mommy, Owen came into my room and took my sweatshirt, and now he won't give it back."

"That's *my* sweatshirt; yours is in the laundry."

"See? I told you. Make him give it back."

"I'm sure you two can work this out. I'm going to mix a pitcher of martinis."

While a diffuse generational boundary gives some parents the illusion that they should settle their children's arguments, a rigid boundary leads other parents to think that they shouldn't even listen to their children's complaints about each other.

Todd burst into the house, shouting, "Goddamn baby!"

Jennifer, two steps behind, was in tears. "Daddy, Todd wouldn't let me ride my bike in the driveway!"

Now what? Ralph didn't mind the swearing so much, but why did the children have to drag him into their fights?

"We were skateboarding. I told her to wait until we were done, but she had to ride her bike right in front of our ramp."

"There wasn't enough room. Besides, you don't own the driveway."

Ralph didn't want to hear any more of this. He was annoyed that the children still expected their parents to settle their arguments. Unlike some people he knew, he didn't intend to intervene, and so he wasn't about to listen. "I'm sorry, but you two will have to settle this yourselves. Now go away and leave me alone."

Jennifer and Todd knew when their father meant business, so they both went up to their rooms. But they didn't settle anything. There was nothing to settle. It was over. There was, in fact, room for both of them on the driveway. What wasn't over was their upset.

What were the children feeling? Ralph didn't have the slightest idea. He never even thought about it.

Todd was upset because Jennifer was always butting in on him and his friends, and he couldn't do anything about it. Mom was always telling him that she was just a little girl and not to pick on her. So how come she was allowed to bother him all the time?

Jennifer was upset because Todd called her a baby in front of his friends. Why did he always have to be so mean? She didn't come to Daddy to ask him to make Todd let her have room to ride her bike; she worked that out for herself. But it's hard to act grown-up with a brother who knows how to torture you and make you cry in front of his friends.

There's such a thing as not enough space, and there's such a thing as too much space. Jennifer and Todd's mother didn't give them enough room to work out their own difficulties. Their father maintained such a rigid boundary between himself and the children that he failed to listen to them when they were upset and needed comforting.

Remember that listening to your children's feelings is different from trying to solve their problems. If Ralph had listened more carefully to his children, he might have realized that although they weren't asking him to settle their disagreement, they were upset. It's never a mistake to listen to a child who is upset. The mistake some parents make is in assuming that it's their responsibility to make their children's upset go away.

Ralph could have spoken to each of his children separately, asked them what happened, and sympathized with their feelings—but without making judgments, taking sides, or trying to settle their dispute.

When it comes to arguments between the children, a clear boundary is firm enough to minimize parental interference in disputes but open enough to encourage listening sympathetically to the children when they're upset. The difference here is between listening to children and trying to control them.

At the beginning of this chapter I said I would discuss some of the questions that parents raise about the application of responsive listening and see what themes emerge. What emerges from this discussion of sibling rivalry is that effective communication with children is a balancing act. On the one hand, it's necessary to be open and understanding, to be available to your children and willing to listen. On the other hand, it's a mistake to be obsessed with controlling your children.

Responsive listening is a tool to help parents cut down on family arguments. But it's a tool that implies a shift in perspective. Whatever else they are, arguments are a struggle for control of a dialogue.

Parents who can't let go, who insist on controlling not just what their children do but also

> **Arguments are driven by two people trying to get their point of view across at the same time. Responsive listening dissolves this struggle by helping parents shift from pressing their case to trying to understand where their children are coming from.**

what they say, will never stop arguing. Responsive listening may be easy to grasp, but to make it work you have to be strong enough to give up control.

"Can I Talk to You about Something?"

As I mentioned previously, interrupting a child who's watching TV to tell her to clean her room raises the question of timing, an issue that turns out to be even more important than you might think in avoiding arguments.

How many of the arguments you have with your children *aren't* predictable? My guess is, not many. If you were willing to take the time to think about it, you could probably write down several instances in the next few days when you and your child are likely to have an argument about something. Here are some typical examples:

- When your child is explaining something and you want to correct him or her.
- When you don't like the way your child speaks to you or to the child's other parent.

- When your children are squabbling.
- When you ask your child to do something that he or she really doesn't want to do.
- When you ask your child about something that he or she thinks of as private.
- When you want to scold your child about not doing some chore.
- When your child wants permission to do something you don't want him or her to do.

If you want to get the most out of this exercise, use these examples as a stimulus to come up with your own list of predictable arguments between you and your child.

Now consider how many of the potential arguments on your list might be prevented by resisting the impulse to say what you feel like saying and, if you still want to have that conversation, choosing a better time and place to initiate it.

———

Tyler and his mother argued constantly about his behavior when he came home from school. No matter how many times she reminded him to change out of his school clothes and do his homework, he never seemed to get around to it. Whenever she spoke to him, he'd say, "Okay, I will." Then when he didn't, and she scolded him, he'd say, "I'm sorry." But nothing changed.

By the time I spoke with Tyler's parents, they were fed up with his behavior and wanted some advice about how to confront him. I thought a confrontation might not be the most effective strategy with a boy who seemed to have trouble putting his feelings into words. So I suggested instead that they write him a note. They agreed to try that idea and decided that Tyler might be more receptive to a note from his father—whom he was less used to putting off.[2]

Here's what they wrote:

———

[2]In many families fathers have an easier time communicating with the children than mothers. That's because mothers get stuck with most of the responsibility for day-to-day managing the children's behavior. There are two lessons here: (1) Most families would be better off with more of a balance in child rearing responsibility, and (2) the less you try to control, the easier it is to communicate with your children.

Dear Tyler,

Mom and I are unhappy because lately we seem to be fighting with you to do all the things you have to do after school. How long would you need to come up with a plan for handling all that you have to do? Twenty-four hours? Two days? We'd like to have a plan you think would work for you, in writing, by the end of the week. The plan needs to include time for homework, changing out of your school clothes, walking the dog, and doing the things you want to do, like playing video games and going on the Internet.

Love,

Dad

To his parents' pleasant surprise, Tyler did indeed come up with a written plan for doing his chores after school, and there were subsequently far fewer arguments.

Some likely-to-be-contentious conversations, of course, are not easily postponed. You can't wait until after supper to tell your child to hurry up and get ready for the school bus. If you don't want your teenager going off with friends without your knowing where and with whom, you can't postpone asking if the friends are at the door.

Here's a related question from a friend of mine.

"Fourteen-year-old Jane comes downstairs dressed for school in a skirt that's too short and a shirt that's too tight. Jane's mom is shocked and says that she can't go to school dressed like that. When Jane demands to know what's wrong with what she's wearing, her mom doesn't know what to say and resorts to 'You look like a hooker'—something her own mother had said to her more than once. What's an example of how she could have used responsive listening instead?"

Obviously it would have been better for this mother not to have told her daughter that she looks like a hooker. But nobody plans to say things like that. They just slip out sometimes. The truth is that if you're not willing to let your son or daughter go to school dressed the way he or she is, the child is going to get upset. No matter what you say, the conversation is going to be unpleasant—and you can't postpone it. All you can do is try to keep it brief.

Here's another example.

A nine-year-old decides to do his parents a favor by mowing the lawn while they're out shopping. His parents come home to find him using the power mower and blow

> **Long conversations are counterproductive and tend to be regarded as punishment. The more you say, the less your children hear.**

up at him about using tools like that when they're not at home. The boy is understandably angry and upset. His parents never explicitly stated this rule but assumed that it was understood. How could they have used responsive listening instead?

By being saints? By not getting upset when their child did something dangerous? I don't know about you, but I'd be upset to come home and find that my child had been doing something as dangerous as using the power mower.

No matter how hard you try to prevent it, there will be times when you say something to make your child upset. Sometimes it may be unavoidable; sometimes you just lose your cool. We all do. While it's useful to learn to do what you can to refrain from triggering reactive responses in your children, it's a mistake to think that you can avoid doing so all the time.

Here's something I learned in my early years of counseling couples. Couples who seek therapy usually fight a lot. Once in therapy, they bring up their fights in sessions.

HE: "She always . . ."

SHE: "That's because he never . . ."

HE: "But that's because she always . . ."

Then the therapist helps them translate their angry attacks into expressions of their underlying, more vulnerable feelings.

"He's a cold son of a bitch" may mean "I'm lonely and feel neglected."

"She's a god-damned shrew" may mean "I feel overwhelmed by her need for more of my time."

Both partners are relieved to resolve the fight, and they're hopeful that from then on they can learn to communicate in a way that avoids fights. Then when, inevitably, they have another fight, maybe a really painful one, they feel totally defeated and helpless. All that progress was an illusion. It's hopeless. They'll *never* learn to get along.

What I discovered is that couples who get discouraged and think they'll never learn to get along are at least partly right. If getting along means avoiding fights, most people never manage to accomplish that.

The trick is to learn to patch things up before too much time passes after a fight. People who don't know how to bury the hatchet after a fight do things like: never apologize—or always apologize; sulk for days; give each other the cold shoulder; always wait for the other person to apologize; and so on. I'm sure you can add to this list—by observing your partner, of course.

The same principle—recognizing the inevitability of a certain number of blowups but learning to be better at resolving them later—applies to parents' arguments with their children.

The secret of resolving arguments later is to use responsive listening. Tell your child that you think you understand what he was trying to say but you're not sure, and then invite him to explain his point of view. But don't just use responsive listening as a gimmick. True responsive listening requires caring enough to pay attention and take an interest in what your child has to say.

Understanding parents don't presume to know their children's thoughts and feelings. Instead, they are open to listening and discovering.

Good-Enough Communication

One of the problems with self-help books[3] is that they feed into the assumption that human nature is endlessly improvable, or, in the case of books on parenting, that being a parent is a skill that can be perfected. Actually, being a parent is an impossible job. We do what we think is right, at least most of the time, and muddle through as best we can. There is, of course, always room for improvement, and my purpose in writing this book was to suggest that parents can improve their commu-

---

[3]This is *not* a self-help book; it is a treatise on the dialectics of intrafamilial communication.

nication with their children by learning to listen responsively. However, while communication between parents and children can be improved, it's a mistake to think that it can be perfected.

Some of you will recognize in the title of this section an echo of psychoanalyst Donald Winnicott's felicitous phrase, "good-enough mothering."[4] Winnicott's point was that while children need a loving environment in which to thrive, this environment needn't be perfect: An *average expectable environment* featuring *good-enough mothering* is sufficient.

The idea that you don't have to be perfect may be familiar, but it bears repeating if it can help lessen the huge burden of guilt most parents place on themselves.

Guilt-ridden parents raise guilt-ridden children.

There are also very practical consequences to parents accepting that they can't endlessly improve their handling of their children. The admirable notion that parents can always do more is rooted in the not-so-admirable notion that parents can ultimately control what happens in their children's lives. Specifically, when it comes to communication, the idea that parents can make things perfect leads to two unfortunate corollaries: that most problems can be prevented and that misunderstandings should always be talked about.

Problems, as you may have noticed, aren't always avoidable. Don't expect that you won't occasionally blow up at your kids, or be late to pick them up, or forget a promise. You may never have told your daughter that she looks like a hooker, but I'm sure we all say and do things as parents that we regret. Don't worry, you'll do it again.

The thing to keep in mind is that we all make mistakes, and so do our kids. You can't prevent misunderstandings or avoid fights, but you can talk about what happened—maybe later, when you both calm down.

One father I know took my advice on patching things up later to heart, and after a particularly unpleasant scene with his son he went back the next day to apologize for overreacting. Here's what he said:

> "I shouldn't have screamed at you like that, but when I repeatedly ask you to shut off the TV and get moving on your homework, and you ignore me, I find it very difficult to control my temper."

---

[4]Winnicott, D. W. (1965). *The maturational process and the facilitating environment.* New York: International Universities Press.

In using the occasion for an apology as an excuse to deliver yet another lecture to his son, this father was doing what we as parents have such a hard time getting away from, and that is the assumption that we're right and our children, when they don't do what we want, are wrong. In this father's "apology" was a metamessage:

> "I'm sorry I acted badly while in charge of you, but it's your fault, and I'm still in charge of telling you what you should and shouldn't do."

Yes, by all means talk with your children about blowups and misunderstandings. But don't insist on your being right and their being wrong.

egocentric (adj.): seeing things only from one's own point of view; having little or no ability to take the other person's perspective into account

---

Sharon was upstairs working at her desk when she heard her daughter Michelle starting down the stairs. "Are you going out?" she called.

"What?" Michelle shouted from the stairs.

"Are you going out?" Sharon repeated, louder.

"I told you," Michelle hollered up in an annoyed voice, "I'm driving over to Naomi's."

"Do you know where my calculator is?" Sharon asked.

"What?" Michelle yelled back.

"Do you know where my calculator is?" Sharon repeated loudly.

"I gave it back to you yesterday!" Michelle shrieked as she went out and slammed the front door.

Sharon was stung by her daughter's tone of voice. *She has no right to talk to me that way,* she thought. *Nobody has a right to talk to me that way. All I did was ask a simple question!* She was seething.

After a couple of minutes, Sharon calmed down and went back to work. When she finished and went downstairs for breakfast she thought about how she might let Michelle know how she didn't appreciate being yelled at like that for asking a simple question. But she also imagined how Michelle might get angry all over again. She seemed to snap at her mother for no good reason at least once a week, and talking to her about it never seemed to do any good.

On further reflection, Sharon could also imagine that Michelle might have gotten annoyed at being shouted at from upstairs when she was on her way out of the house. And she'd said more than once how annoying it was that Sharon often forgot things she'd told her. Would talking about what happened do any good? Maybe Sharon should just let it go?

———————

That would be my advice. What would be the point of this mother telling her daughter that she didn't like being spoken to in a nasty tone of voice? Is that news to anyone? Some people get angry when provoked. If you live with such a person, you have to expect a certain amount of that. Sharon could of course tell Michelle that she felt bad when Michelle spoke that way to her. She could also find out what had made Michelle so annoyed. Was it being shouted at when she was on her way out of the house? Was it that her mother didn't remember things she told her? Was it that she felt wrongly accused of failing to return her mother's calculator?

Sharon could try to talk to Michelle about any or all of these things, but what really would be the point? Would it be different from a parent trying to control every interaction with her child? Even if Sharon asked Michelle why she was annoyed, wouldn't her real aim be to give her daughter a lecture on not being rude? One more question. Even assuming that Michelle may have been annoyed at her mother for any or all of the reasons suggested here, do you doubt that she knew she had spoken rudely to her mother and, at least to some extent, felt bad about doing so?

———————

In many ways Patrick was a good kid. He did his homework faithfully, didn't mind helping out around the house, and was often a genuine pleasure to be with. But he had one habit that drove his father absolutely crazy. No matter how many times Ray reminded him, Patrick never put his dirty dishes in the sink. He always left whatever plate or bowl he used on the living room couch.

Ray tried reminding Patrick gently, tried having long talks with him and explaining why it bothered him so much when he left his dirty dishes around. Ray even tried asking Patrick if there was a reason he didn't put his dishes away. No matter what his father said or did, Patrick always apologized for leaving his dishes out; but it never seemed to do any good. He'd do the same thing again next time. He just didn't seem to remember, or, if he did, didn't seem to care enough to stop doing it.

What to do? Ray has three choices. He can do what most parents do—continue to nag his son, with varying amounts of patience and exasperation. He could punish the boy severely and consistently enough to change his behavior. Or he could let it go. Decide that although he really hated his son's leaving dirty dishes on the couch, and didn't want him to grow up to be an inconsiderate person, it wasn't worth having all these unpleasant interactions with his son to keep bugging him about the dishes.

What rules you as a parent decide to enforce and what you decide to let go is, of course, up to you. What I'm suggesting is that there are many problems that aren't going to be solved by being talking about.

How do you decide that talking about a particular issue may not be useful? Should a mother, for example, talk to her daughter about the daughter's nasty tone with her? Should a father talk with his son about the boy's failure to carry his dirty dishes into the kitchen? My advice is to ask yourself this: Have you had this conversation before? Did it do any good?

Wait a minute! All of a sudden I'm telling you that talking things over may not help? Wasn't the whole point of this book to enable parents to transform arguments with their children into productive conversations? Yes, but. . . .

Yes, the point of this book was to help parents learn to cut down on arguments with their kids. *But* the secret of doing so involves not just practicing a particular skill—responsive listening; that skill turns out to be based on an underlying shift in the dynamics of a parent's relationship with his or her children. The shift I'm talking about is from the parent's perspective to the child's. Listening responsively involves a specific application of this shift—from repeating what you have to say to listening to what your child has to say. But the shift is more than that. It's a shift from staying stuck inside your own perspective to learning to take your child's perspective. Frankly, it's not an easy shift to make.

INDEX

ABOUT THE AUTHOR

Michael P. Nichols, PhD, Professor of Psychology at the College of William and Mary (Williamsburg, Virginia), is the author of *The Lost Art of Listening, No Place to Hide,* and *Family Healing* (with Salvador Minuchin), among other books. He is a popular speaker and has been a guest on numerous television programs. In addition to teaching and practicing family therapy, Dr. Nichols is a national masters powerlifting champion.